Bipolar Depression

Editor

JOHN L. BEYER

PSYCHIATRIC CLINICS
OF NORTH AMERICA

www.psych.theclinics.com

March 2016 • Volume 39 • Number 1

ELSEVIER

1600 John F. Kennedy Boulevard • Suite 1800 • Philadelphia, Pennsylvania, 19103-2899

http://www.theclinics.com

PSYCHIATRIC CLINICS OF NORTH AMERICA Volume 39, Number 1
March 2016 ISSN 0193-953X, ISBN-13: 978-0-323-41661-0

Editor: Lauren Boyle
Developmental Editor: Kristen Helm

Psychiatric Clinics of North America (ISSN 0193-953X) is published quarterly by Elsevier Inc., 360 Park Avenue South, New York, NY 10010-1710. Months of issue are March, June, September, and December. Business and Editorial Offices: 1600 John F. Kennedy Blvd., Suite 1800, Philadelphia, PA 19103-2899. Periodicals postage paid at New York, NY and additional mailing offices. Subscription prices are $300.00 per year (US individuals), $598.00 per year (US institutions), $100.00 per year (US students/residents), $365.00 per year (Canadian individuals), $455.00 per year (international individuals), $753.00 per year (Canadian & international institutions), and $220.00 per year (Canadian & international students/residents). Foreign air speed delivery is included in all *Clinics'* subscription prices. All prices are subject to change without notice. **POSTMASTER:** Send address changes to *Psychiatric Clinics of North America,* Elsevier Health Sciences Division, Subscription Customer Service, 3251 Riverport Lane, Maryland Heights, MO 63043. **Customer Service: 1-800-654-2452 (US). From outside the United States, call 1-314-447-8871. Fax: 1-314-447-8029. E-mail: journalscustomerservice-usa@elsevier.com (for print support) and journalsonline support-usa@elsevier.com (for online support).**

Reprints. For copies of 100 or more, of articles in this publication, please contact the Commercial Reprints Department, Elsevier Inc., 360 Park Avenue South, New York, New York 10010-1710. Tel.: 212-633-3874, Fax: 212-633-3820, E-mail: reprints@elsevier.com.

Psychiatric Clinics of North America is covered in *MEDLINE/PubMed (Index Medicus), Current Contents/Social and Behavioral Sciences, Social Science Citation Index, Embase/Excerpta Medica,* and PsycINFO.

Contributors

EDITOR

JOHN L. BEYER, MD
Professor of Psychiatry; Director, Mood Disorder Clinic, Duke University Medical Center, Duke South Clinics, Durham, North Carolina

AUTHORS

JOHN L. BEYER, MD
Professor of Psychiatry; Director, Mood Disorder Clinic, Duke University Medical Center, Duke South Clinics, Durham, North Carolina

DRUE CLARK, PharmD, BCACP
Clinical Pharmacist, Mission Health Outpatient Clinical Pharmacy Services, Asheville, North Carolina

AMY K. CUELLAR, PhD
Team Leader, Michael E. DeBakey VA Medical Center; Assistant Professor, Menninger Department of Psychiatry and Behavioral Sciences, Baylor College of Medicine, Houston, Texas

COLIN A. DEPP, PhD
Department of Psychiatry, UC San Diego, La Jolla, California; Desert-Pacific Mental Illness Research, Education, and Clinical Center, VA San Diego Healthcare System, San Diego, California

SHEENA DEV, BS
Department of Psychiatry, UC San Diego, La Jolla, California; SDSU-UCSD Joint Doctoral Program, Clinical Psychology, San Diego, California

LISA T. EYLER, PhD
Associate Professor, Department of Psychiatry, UC San Diego, La Jolla, California; Desert-Pacific Mental Illness Research, Education, and Clinical Center, VA San Diego Healthcare System, San Diego, California

ANDA GERSHON, PhD
Instructor, Department of Psychiatry and Behavioral Sciences, Stanford University, Stanford, California

FERNANDO S. GOES, MD
Department of Psychiatry and Behavioral Sciences, Johns Hopkins University School of Medicine, Baltimore, Maryland

NATHANIEL R. HERR, PhD
Assistant Professor, Department of Psychology, American University, Washington, DC

NICOLAS HOERTEL, MD, MPH
Department of Psychiatry, Chef de Clinique des Universités-Assistant des Hôpitaux, Corentin Celton Hospital, Assistance Publique-Hôpitaux de Paris (APHP); INSERM UMR 894, Psychiatry and Neurosciences Center, Issy-les-Moulineaux, France; PRES Sorbonne Paris Cité, Paris Descartes University, Paris, France

SHERI L. JOHNSON, PhD
Professor and Director of the Cal Mania (CALM) Program, Department of Psychology, University of California Berkeley, Berkeley, California

ROGER S. McINTYRE, MD, FRCPC
Head, Mood Disorder Psychopharmacology Unit, University Health Network; Professor of Psychiatry and Pharmacology, University of Toronto, Toronto, Ontario, Canada

KIBBY McMAHON, BA
Cognitive-Behavioral Research and Treatment Program, Graduate Student, Department of Psychology and Neuroscience, Duke University Medical Center, Durham, North Carolina

ANDREW J. MUZYK, PharmD
Associate Professor, Campbell University College of Pharmacy and Health Sciences, Buies Creek, North Carolina

ANDRADA D. NEACSIU, PhD
Cognitive-Behavioral Research and Treatment Program, Assistant Professor, Department of Psychiatry and Behavioral Sciences, Duke University Medical Center, Durham, North Carolina

MARTHA E. PAYNE, PhD, RD, MPH
Research Development Associate, Office of Research Development; Office of the Dean, Duke University School of Medicine, Durham, North Carolina

ROY H. PERLIS, MD, MSc
Director, Center for Experimental Drugs and Diagnostics, Massachusetts General Hospital; Associate Professor, Department of Psychiatry, Harvard Medical School, Boston, Massachusetts

ROBERT M. POST, MD
Professor of Psychiatry, George Washington School of Medicine, Washington, DC; Bipolar Collaborative Network, Bethesda, Maryland

JOSHUA D. ROSENBLAT, MD
Resident of Psychiatry, Clinician Scientist Stream, University of Toronto, Toronto, Ontario, Canada

PAUL A. VÖHRINGER, MD, MSc, MPH
Research Assistant Professor, Department of Psychiatry, Tufts University School of Medicine, Boston, Massachusetts; Assistant Professor of Psychiatry, University of Chile, Santiago, Chile

MARLA F. WALD, MD
Assistant Professor, Department of Psychiatry and Behavioral Sciences, Duke University Medical Center, Durham, North Carolina

RICHARD H. WEISLER, MD
Adjunct Associate Professor of Psychiatry, Duke University Medical Center, Durham, North Carolina; Adjunct Professor of Psychiatry, University of North Carolina School of Medicine, Chapel Hill, North Carolina

NOGA ZERUBAVEL, PhD
Cognitive-Behavioral Research and Treatment Program, Assistant Professor, Department of Psychiatry and Behavioral Sciences, Duke University Medical Center, Durham, North Carolina

Contents

> Rates of misdiagnosis between major depressive disorder and bipolar disorder have been reported to be substantial, and the consequence of such misdiagnosis is likely to be a delay in achieving effective control of symptoms, in some cases spanning many years. Particularly in the midst of a depressive episode, or early in the illness course, it may be challenging to distinguish the 2 mood disorders purely on the basis of cross-sectional features. To date, no useful biological markers have been reliably shown to distinguish between bipolar disorder and major depressive disorder.

> Bipolar depression is the most common and difficult-to-treat phase of bipolar disorder. Antidepressants for unipolar depression are among the most widely used drugs, but recent data and meta-analyses indicate a lack of efficacy. Many of the drugs discussed here are graded provisionally for the strength of the findings in the literature, safety and tolerability, and likely utility of use in patients with bipolar disorder. Successful long-term treatment of bipolar depression is critical to preventing illness-related morbidity, disability, cognitive decline, suicide, and premature loss of years of life expectancy largely from the excess medical mortality associated with cardiovascular disorders.

> The gold standard for treating bipolar depression is based on the combination of mood stabilizers and psychotherapy. Therefore, the authors present evidence-based models and promising approaches for psychotherapy for bipolar depression. Cognitive-behavioral therapy, family focused therapy, interpersonal and social rhythm therapy, mindfulness-based cognitive therapy, and dialectical behavior therapy are discussed. Behavioral activation, the cognitive behavioral analysis system of psychotherapy, and the unified protocol as promising future directions are presented. This review informs medical providers of the most appropriate referral guidelines for psychotherapy for bipolar depression. The authors conclude with a decision tree delineating optimal referrals to each psychotherapy approach.

Medication management of bipolar depression in pregnancy and lactation is best done by assessing each patient's and family's needs in detail. Keeping pregnant patients as psychiatrically stable as possible is the most important principle for clinicians. Unfortunately, there is no risk-free situation for patients with psychiatric illness. This is often the most difficult and hard to accept reality for these patients, families, and clinicians. Clinicians serve these patients best by being as transparent as possible about the risk/benefit analysis of each patient's situation with the realization that ultimately the decisions are made by the patient and family.

As with physical conditions, bipolar disorder is likely to be impacted by diet and nutrition. Patients with bipolar disorder have been noted to have relatively unhealthy diets, which may in part be the reason they also have an elevated risk of metabolic syndrome and obesity. An improvement in the quality of the diet should improve a bipolar patient's overall health risk profile, but it may also improve their psychiatric outcomes. New insights into biological dysfunctions that may be present in bipolar disorder have presented new theoretic frameworks for understanding the relationship between diet and bipolar disorder.

A growing body of research suggests that the social environment exerts a powerful influence on the course of bipolar depression. This article reviews longitudinal research to suggest that trauma, negative life events, social support deficits, and family difficulties are common and predict a more severe course of depression when present among those diagnosed with bipolar disorder. The triggers of bipolar depression overlap with those documented for unipolar depression, suggesting that many of the treatment targets for unipolar depression may be applicable for bipolar depression.

Depression and cognitive impairment are pervasive and highly disabling aspects of bipolar disorder. Although cognitive impairment is partially independent from mood episodes, depressive symptoms may increase the risk of cognitive impairment in bipolar disorder through inflammatory processes as well as health risks such as obesity and sedentary behavior. Novel treatment avenues at the intersection of bipolar depression and cognitive impairment target inflammation directly or indirectly health behaviors such as diet, physical activity, and sleep hygiene.

Suicide behaviors (ideation, attempts, and completions) are unfortunately common in patients with bipolar disorder. It is estimated that 25 to 50% attempt suicide at least once during their lifetime, and 6% to 19% complete suicide. Risk factors include a family history of suicide, previous suicide attempts, younger age of onset, comorbid psychiatric illnesses, and psychological constructs like hopelessness. Pharmacologic treatment may impact suicidal behaviors, either increasing vulnerability or resilience. Clinicians need to be particularly sensitive to their patient's thoughts and beliefs about death, particularly during stressful times of life or when in a depressive/mixed episode of bipolar disorder.

The pathophysiology of bipolar disorder (BD) remains poorly understood. Current psychopharmacologic treatments are often poorly tolerated and carry high rates of treatment resistance. Mounting evidence has suggested that innate immune system dysfunction may play a role in the pathophysiology of BD. Elevated proinflammatory cytokine levels have been identified. The innate immune system is a novel therapeutic target in BD. Lithium has been shown to have antiinflammatory properties. Further research is needed to establish the role of antiinflammatory agents in the treatment of BD; however, evidence from several clinical trials indicates that antiinflammatory agents may be incorporated into clinical practice soon.

Although genetic studies of bipolar disorder (BD) have been pursued for decades, it has only been in the last several years that clearly replicated findings have emerged. These findings, typically of modest effects, point to a polygenic genetic architecture consisting of multiple common and rare susceptibility variants. While larger genome-wide association studies are ongoing, the advent of whole exome and genome sequencing should lead to the identification of rare, and potentially more penetrant, variants. Progress along both fronts will provide novel insights into the biology of BD and help usher in a new era of personalized medicine and improved treatments.

PSYCHIATRIC CLINICS OF NORTH AMERICA

FORTHCOMING ISSUES

June 2016
Schizophrenia: Advances and Current
Management
Peter F. Buckley, *Editor*

September 2016
Psychopharmacotherapeutic Side Effects
Rajnish Mago, *Editor*

December 2016
Violence
James L. Knoll, *Editor*

RECENT ISSUES

December 2015
Sleep Disorders and Mental Health
Andrew Winokur and Jayesh Kamath,
Editors

September 2015
Clinical Psychiatry: Recent Advances and
Future Directions
David A. Baron and Lawrence S. Gross,
Editors

June 2015
Young-Onset Dementias
Chiadi U. Onyike, *Editor*

RELATED INTEREST

Medical Clinics of North America, September 2014 (Vol. 98, No. 5)
Psychiatric Diagnosis and Management in Primary Care
Genevieve L. Pagalilauan, *Editor*
Available at: http://www.medical.theclinics.com/

THE CLINICS ARE AVAILABLE ONLINE!
Access your subscription at:
www.theclinics.com

Preface

The Challenge of Bipolar Depression in the 21st Century

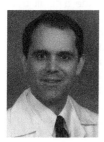

John L. Beyer, MD
Editor

For a young psychiatrist starting practice over a quarter century ago, diagnosing and treating bipolar disorder appeared simplistically easy. Step 1: Is the patient manic? Step 2: Treat with lithium. Step 3?

There really was no step 3.

However, for all experienced clinicians who have treated patients over time, and for all patients with bipolar disorder who have struggled to maintain their emotional stability over time, there must be a step 3, and a step 4, step 5, 6, 7, and more.

In 1995, an expert treatment algorithm for bipolar depression consisted of only one treatment decision: lithium or lithium + antidepressant. After that was a large question mark.[1] In the last 20 years, great strides have been made in the understanding and treatment of bipolar disorder; and although there have been over 15 medications approved by the FDA for the treatment of some part of bipolar disorder, only three (olanzapine/fluoxetine combination, quetiapine/quetiapine XR, lurasidone) have actually been approved for the treatment of bipolar depression. Thus, for the most common mood state in bipolar disorder, our list of proven therapies remains discouragingly small and our understanding of the condition is limited.

Part of our problem has been in our diagnostic focus. To be bipolar, we thought, was to be manic. However, we have come to realize that for most of our patients, it is not the manias that define bipolar disorder, but the depressions. In fact, bipolar patients will have more than three episodes of depression for every manic episode, and since depressive episodes last much longer than manic episodes, they will spend a proportionally greater amount of time suffering with their depressive symptoms. Yet research into the treatment of bipolar depression has sadly lagged behind treatment research for both the manic phase of bipolar disorder and the similar symptomed but etiologically different unipolar depression.

This is the challenge of bipolar depression.

Psychiatr Clin N Am 39 (2016) xi–xii
http://dx.doi.org/10.1016/j.psc.2015.11.001
0193-953X/16/$ – see front matter © 2016 Elsevier Inc. All rights reserved.

This issue focuses on bipolar depression and our current understanding of the disease. In our first article, Drs Vöhringer and Perlis discuss the differentiation of bipolar disorder from unipolar depression. After this, there are four articles dealing with issues surrounding treatment of bipolar depression. First, Dr Post turns his attention and considerable clinical and research experience to a discussion of rational pharmacologic treatment. Second, Dr McMahon and colleagues review psychotherapeutic options for bipolar depression. Third, Dr Wald and colleagues review the difficult but common experience of treating bipolar depressed patients who are pregnant. Finally, Drs Beyer and Payne review the role of nutrition in the treatment of bipolar depression.

There are then a series of articles focusing on issues with which patients with bipolar depression struggle. Dr Johnson and colleagues discuss the influence of trauma and social support in bipolar depression. Dr Depp and colleagues then discuss cognitive changes associated with bipolar depression. Drs Beyer and Weisler discuss the problem of suicide and bipolar depression. Drs Rosenblat and McIntyre review the possible role that inflammation may have in bipolar disorder. Finally, Dr Goes reviews our current understanding of genetics in bipolar disorder.

As I reflect over the last quarter century, I am pleased to know we have advanced our understanding of bipolar disorder. However, as this issue illustrates, it is in the depressive episodes that we may find both the humanity of our patients and our humility before this illness. This is the challenge of bipolar depression.

John L. Beyer, MD
Duke University Medical Center
Box 3519 DUMC
Room 4082B, Yellow Zone
Duke South Clinics
Durham, NC 27710, USA

E-mail address:
john.beyer@dm.duke.edu

REFERENCE

1. Suppes T, Calabrese JR, Mitchell PB, et al. Algorithms for the treatment of bipolar manic-depressive illness. Psychopharmacol Bull 1995;31(3):469–74.

Discriminating Between Bipolar Disorder and Major Depressive Disorder

Paul A. Vöhringer, MD, MSc, MPH[a,b], Roy H. Perlis, MD, MSc[c,*]

KEYWORDS

- Diagnosis • Nosology • Misdiagnosis • Bipolar disorder • Major depressive disorder
- Irritability

KEY POINTS

- During depressive episodes, bipolar disorder (BD) and major depressive disorder may be difficult to distinguish.
- Misdiagnosis may lead to delay in effective treatment and to exposure to ineffective treatment.
- Illness features more often observed in BD may include psychomotor slowing or agitation, cognitive impairment, mood lability, psychosis, onset in the peripartum period, and early age at illness onset, among others, but none is sufficient to warrant a bipolar diagnosis.
- Only a careful, systematic assessment for current or past manic or hypomanic symptoms allows accurate diagnosis.
- Biomarkers useful in distinguishing the 2 mood disorders have not yet been established.

Despite decades of effort, psychiatry still lacks a reliable biological marker to distinguish the 2 depressive disorders, major depressive disorder (MDD) and bipolar disorder (BD), whose phenomenology can be extremely similar. There remain 2 commonly held assumptions about these 2 disorders. The first assumption is that MDD and BD are clear-cut and easily separable diagnostic conditions, requiring only careful assessment to distinguish. The second assumption is that there is no true difference in the clinical phenomenology of unipolar depression (UD) versus bipolar depression, and that, at least in the midst of a depressive episode, the 2 disorders cannot be distinguished. Unfortunately, both assumptions likely oversimplify the evidence base and tend to inhibit rigorous investigation by introducing biased assessment. The oft-cited observation

[a] Department of Psychiatry, Tufts University School of Medicine, 800 Washington Street, Boston, MA 02111, USA; [b] Department of Psychiatry, University of Chile, Av. Independencia 1027, Santiago 8071146, Chile; [c] Department of Psychiatry, Center for Experimental Drugs and Diagnostics, Massachusetts General Hospital, Harvard Medical School, 185 Cambridge Street, Boston, MA 02114, USA
* Corresponding author.
E-mail address: rperlis@mgh.harvard.edu

Psychiatr Clin N Am 39 (2016) 1–10
http://dx.doi.org/10.1016/j.psc.2015.10.001
0193-953X/16/$ – see front matter © 2016 Elsevier Inc. All rights reserved.

psych.theclinics.com

that approximately one-third of individuals may wait 10 years or more for an accurate diagnosis can be challenged on numerous levels, but the fundamental point that patients are ill-served by the current diagnostic system is hard to dispute.

Despite the fact that MDD and BP are both included in the same group of conditions called mood disorders, clinical distinctions between them have been recognized for many decades.[1] Although clinically distinct, bipolar depression, and more specifically, the depressive phase of bipolar type II (BPII), has proven especially difficult to differentiate from MDD. Both have been defined mainly by the presence of depressive symptoms, and Diagnostic and Statistical Manual of Mental Disorders (DSM)-5 continues the approach of prior editions in defining criteria for depressive episodes that are identical across these 2 disorders.[2] Furthermore, as most patients with BPII present for treatment when depressed rather than hypomanic, it is not surprising that it is difficult to differentiate cross-sectionally between BPII and UD.[3]

MOTIVATION FOR DISCRIMINATING BIPOLAR DISORDER FROM MAJOR DEPRESSIVE DISORDER

If the presentations are so similar, why bother to differentiate? Could this represent an example of the much-maligned notion of pseudo-specificity, carving biology at joints that do not necessarily even exist? For some clinicians and health systems, the drive to distinguish is administrative: billing requires a diagnostic code, either MDD or BD, which may account for the striking frequency of "not otherwise specified" diagnoses. However, at the core, there are 2 key reasons it might be worthwhile to distinguish BD from MDD, and importantly, they suggest potentially different solutions. To begin with, the diagnosis may have predictive validity: it may convey important information about prospective course. In particular, it may convey information about probable treatment response: interventions for the 2 disorders may be almost totally different. Generally speaking, BD requires attention to treating and preventing manic/hypomanic episodes (and to not inadvertently worsening or precipitating such episodes), whereas MDD treatment can focus solely on depressive symptoms and prevention of depressions. A second, less commonly appreciated reason is the need to draw such a distinction to facilitate biological investigation. That is, distinguishing the 2 disorders more effectively would facilitate the identification of associated biology, whereas high rates of misclassification might make such studies infeasible.

Absence of Antidepressant Efficacy

There is solid if not entirely consistent evidence suggesting lack of efficacy, or at least more modest efficacy, for antidepressants (the most common drug used in both conditions[4]), specifically in bipolar depression. Recently, new evidence supporting this small effect has emerged: 2 randomized clinical trials (RCT), double-blinded, testing "modern" antidepressants added to mood stabilizers, compared with placebo, showed neither acute nor long-term efficacy for bipolar patients suffering from a depressive episode.[5,6] In addition, a meta-analysis included these already mentioned 2 RCT along with 4 more RCT (around 1300 patients total) and showed an acute modest effect of antidepressants when added to mood stabilizers or atypical antipsychotics, but greater risk for manic episodes over a year of follow-up.[7]

On the other hand, there is robust evidence suggesting antidepressants' efficacy for MDD. Large, well-developed, and funded by National Institutes of Health, clinical trials, such as STAR-D, have found that almost two-thirds of UD patients have reached clinical remission in a year period of treatment.[8] In addition, a recent reanalysis of a meta-analysis purporting to show that antidepressants lack efficacy compared with placebo[9] actually showed that these drugs are in fact efficacious in moderate and severe depressive episodes, albeit less so in mild ones.[10]

Risk for Antidepressant-Associated Mania

The meta-analytic results introduce the important notion that treatments used for MDD may actually worsen the long-term course of illness in BP disorders, resulting in increasing risk for manic episodes or simply more frequent mood episodes, or cycle acceleration.[11] In fact, antidepressant-induced mania is substantially more common in bipolar than in UD, occurring in about 20% to 50% of persons with BD,[12,13] versus less than 1% in persons with UD, as reported in the STAR-D study.[11] (Of course, this comparison can be misleading: if one becomes manic, regardless of precipitant, it can be argued that the true diagnosis is BD; the subsequent longitudinal course in these individuals remains understudied.)

Another concern with antidepressant use among BP individuals is the possibility of precipitating or exacerbating mixed (manic) symptoms during depressive episodes.[14,15] Because mixed symptoms or states are associated with increases in suicidality in some studies, at least some proportion of antidepressant-induced suicidality in children and adults[16,17] may actually represent the induction of mixed states by antidepressants in individuals with undetected BD.

Although the risk of MDD diagnosis among BP individuals is typically emphasized in reviews, it should be noted that the opposite—incorrect assignment of BP among individuals who truly have MDD—may also have substantial consequences.[18,19] In lieu of antidepressants, such individuals may instead receive pharmacotherapies known to be ineffective or modestly effective in MDD (lithium monotherapy, lamotrigine, for example) or those with substantial toxicity and poorer tolerability (second-generation antipsychotics, for example) when safer options exist.

PREVALENCE AND CONTRIBUTORS TO MISDIAGNOSIS

As the consequences described in the previous section suggest, a particular problem may be misdiagnosis of BD as MDD. BPII is more commonly misdiagnosed as recurrent MDD.[20,21] When a true bipolar patient is assessed in a depressive phase, there is a relative risk of more than 40% of being mistakenly diagnosed as MDD.[22] Other studies have suggested that up to half of patients with recurrent depressive episodes may in fact suffer from BPII.[23] On the other hand, evidence from unselected depressive cohorts who have undergone minimal screening suggests these risks may be profoundly inflated: among ~4000 individuals in STAR*D who presented in a depressive episode and were screened only to exclude obvious prior manic episodes, a very small minority subsequently exhibited mania.[11] This finding persisted even among individuals with greater degrees of prospectively established treatment resistance.

Misdiagnosis may occur in part due to a lack of complaints from patients experiencing milder mood elevation or periods of time whereby they were functioning better than usual.[24] Clinicians themselves may also play a crucial role in misdiagnosis of BD, when they do not adequately ask for prior histories of hypomania (using broad screening questions) from the patient and, perhaps more importantly, close relatives or friends. In fact, reliability of diagnosis can improve up to 16% with specific strategies used to address previous hypomanic episodes.[25]

One patient survey suggested individuals with BD may wait up to 10 years for this diagnosis. During this time, patients on average see 8 clinicians and receive antidepressant treatments at least 4 times.[20] A key caveat here is that initial episodes may simply be depressive in nature, that is, much of this delay may be accounted for because manic or hypomanic symptoms have simply not yet occurred, and clinicians simply cannot know what the future holds.[26]

Individuals with BPII may be also misdiagnosed as having other clinical conditions such as borderline personality disorder (BPD),[27] anxiety disorder,[23] or adjustment disorder.[28] Particularly in the case of anxiety disorders, such diagnosis may be rendered more complex by the very high rates of comorbidity between BPD and anxiety[29]; that is, both diagnoses may be correct. In the specific case of distinguishing between bipolar and borderline, several differences may be relevant: if patients have history of sexual or physical trauma, self-mutilation, or dissociative symptoms, BPD may be more likely. Conversely, if patients have a family history of mood illness and marked episodic psychomotor activation, in the absence of sexual trauma and self-mutilation, a borderline diagnosis may be less likely.[30]

Finally, clinician biases, conscious or unconscious, may also contribute to misdiagnosis. For example, in general, conferring a BD diagnosis entails greater work for the physician in terms of patient education and medication management. In cases where the precise diagnosis is in question, it may be tempting to default to the one easier to describe and manage. Conversely, more than a decade of pharmaceutical industry-sponsored continuing medical education about the dangers of underrecognition of BD may lead clinicians to overestimate the prior probability that a presenting patient has BD, particularly when initial antidepressant treatments have been ineffective or poorly tolerated.

STRATEGIES FOR IMPROVING DIAGNOSIS

Clinicians who seek a single rating scale or group of clinical features that reliably distinguish BD from MDD during the depressive phase of illness are likely to be disappointed, despite the proliferation of rating scales, medical education efforts, and reviews purporting to allow just that. The only convincing strategy for improving diagnostic accuracy is to focus on longitudinal assessments of patients, rather than relying solely on the single, cross-sectional symptomatic approach used in many clinical contexts. As Kraepelin wrote, "Diagnosis is prognosis,"[31] by which he meant that an accurate psychiatric diagnosis requires consideration of the longitudinal course of illness. To begin with, BD patients tend to experience disease symptoms early in their life. A retrospective assessment of a large adult cohort indicated that approximately one-third of BD patients experienced symptom onset before age 13, and another approximately one-third experienced symptom onset between the ages of 13 and 18.[26] In many cases, an initial psychiatric diagnosis is conferred during school years; most frequently, initial diagnosis is attention deficit disorder, anxiety disorders, or behavioral disturbances.[32] These patients are likely to receive psychotropic drugs as well, because multiple severe symptomatic episodes are commonly described.[32] Likewise, more frequent recurrence is also associated with greater risk for BD than MDD in multiple studies.[33]

More generally, age at first episode is among the clinical features most reliably associated with BD risk, with mean and median onset age consistently younger in BD compared with MDD individuals.[34–37] There is not, however, a clear-cut point to facilitate diagnosis. Rather, the younger the onset of mood episodes, the greater should the concern be for a bipolar course.

Gender distribution of mood disorders also represents an area of difference between MDD and BD. The differentiation of MDD from BPII may be especially relevant, because women suffer these disorders more frequently than men.[38] Lifetime prevalence of MDD is reported to be 16.6%; however, women are twice as likely as men to experience this disorder.[39] BPII is substantially less common than MDD, with reported lifetime prevalence in the United States of 1.1%.[40] Nevertheless, BPII may be more prevalent in women than men as well.[41] (In particular, severe postpartum mood episodes may be particularly common among women with BD.[42])

A large body of evidence also reflects efforts to distinguish MDD from BD based on nosology. Although DSM-5 diagnostic criteria for major depressive episodes in the context of MDD and BD are identical, as in prior DSM editions, other results suggest subtle differences in symptoms. Selected clinical features observed more often in MDD or BD are summarized in **Table 1**. A large study of mood disorders by Mitchell and colleagues[43] found higher rates of psychomotor retardation, greater difficulty with cognition, more early morning awakening, more pronounced worsening of morning mood, and more frequent psychotic symptoms in bipolar depression relative to UD. Another often-cited feature is irritability, which may be an indicator of manic or mixed episodes; it bears noting that such irritable periods of elevation are at least as common as euphoric manias.[1] One study suggested that irritability, in the form of paniclike "anger attacks," is found more frequently in BD than UD.[44]

Other studies also suggest subtle differences between symptom profiles across disorders. For instance, atypical neurovegetative symptoms (hypersomnia and hyperphagia) may be more prevalent in BDII depressive episodes.[45] Another study showed that when compared with MDD, BDII patients had more prevalent suicidality and higher levels of psychomotor restlessness and agitation.[35]

BIOMARKERS AND BIOLOGY

Consideration of family and twin studies provides insight into the extent to which biomarkers might distinguish MDD from BP. In general, studies of twins suggest substantially greater concordance among monozygotic twins for BD compared with MDD; although both disorders are heritable, BP is substantially more so. In family studies, having a first-degree family member with BD increases the risk to the proband of BP by ~7-fold. However, importantly, risk is also increased albeit less so for MDD.

Table 1
Selected clinical features favoring bipolar disorder or major depressive disorder reported in at least one published study

Tension/fearfulness	BD > MDD
Somatic complaints	MDD > BD
Psychomotor agitation	BD > MDD
Atypical depressive features	BD > MDD
Depressive mixed states	BD > MDD
Irritability	BD > MDD
Psychotic features	BD > MDD
Postpartum onset	BD > MDD
Early age at illness onset (ie, before age 25)	BD > MDD
Pain sensitivity	MDD > BD
Appetite loss	MDD > BD
Insomnia (initial)	MDD > BD
Insomnia (late)	BD > MDD
Mood lability within episode	BD > MDD

Taken together, these lines of investigation going back many decades indicate what will be apparent to any clinician who has generated an extended pedigree for a patient with BD: although BP runs in families, these families often manifest other psychopathology, including MDD. As such, simply concluding that a family history of BP predicts BP overlooks the substantially greater prevalence of MDD and may contribute to misdiagnosis. (For further discussion, see[46].) Put another way, clinicians already have a biomarker for BP, albeit a very imperfect one, and already this biomarker is applied inaccurately.

A major challenge in identifying biomarkers is the absence of a useful gold standard for BPII. Reliability of this diagnosis in DSM-5 is even worse than prior editions; so poor that even finding this value in the field trial publication is nontrivial. Therefore, any study trying to find biology that distinguishes MDD from BPII must contend with the limitations of the gold standard, rendering studies that report near-perfect discrimination highly suspect.

Another challenge in biomarker studies seeking to discriminate MDD from BPII is the obstacles posed by considering trait versus state. Features associated with BP—differences in treatment, greater probability of depression at any given time, perhaps greater overall severity of depression—may readily confound an apparent biomarker. Although this is obvious if medications are considered directly (for example, stating that lithium treatment predicts bipolarity), it may be less so when medication or symptom proxies are considered instead (for example, finding that poorer renal function or oral glucose tolerance predicts bipolarity, or that greater levels of HPA axis activity associated with stress or treatment effects).

Perhaps the greatest risk in interpreting this burgeoning literature, though, arises from the problem of overfitting.[47] When a sufficient number of predictors are considered, it should be possible to discriminate 2 subsets with near-perfect accuracy in a single data set. Unfortunately, these predictors may be substantially less useful in other data sets; the estimates in the initial data are thus referred to as optimistic, an ironic turn of phrase insofar as authors remain ever optimistic when they present their biomarker panels in print. The solution for this limitation is straightforward but hard: putative biomarkers require testing in additional cohorts to estimate their performance, ideally ones as representative of the target population as possible.

With these caveats in mind, a growing number of biomarkers have been reported to distinguish BP and MDD, although none has been replicated consistently. One recent report described predictive differences in a panel of urine metabolites, for example.[48] Although numerous blood biomarkers have also been reported, these are more often examined in contrasts between BP and healthy controls, when the key comparison would be BP and MDD.[49] The body of work distinguishes groups of individuals with BP and MDD on the basis of neuroimaging, and the challenges in extrapolating from these group differences to individual diagnosis have also been recently reviewed.[50]

LIMITATIONS AND NEXT STEPS

As with biomarkers, the published literature on clinical discrimination of these disorders also suffers from some major limitations impeding utility. To begin with, most studies examine relatively selected populations and use a case-control, rather than a cohort, design. For example, a common strategy is to contrast individuals diagnosed in one setting to individuals diagnosed in another.[37] Even when all individuals come from a single setting, unblinded assessors may inadvertently introduce confirmation bias: a mood disorder program where family history of BD represents a strong hypothesized predictor of BD will be more likely to confer that diagnosis in individuals with such a family history, thereby increasing an apparent correlation. Furthermore, the most frequent comparison when differentiating BD from MDD has relied on BDI populations.[37,51] There is scant current evidence from BDII clinical population, despite the fact that these patients seem to be more prevalent than BDI individuals.[33,40]

As such, few studies directly inform the clinical problem at hand, namely, how to approach an individual patient who presents in the midst of a depressive episode and without clear-cut evidence of a prior manic episode. Although the results summarized above are intriguing, the extent to which they generalize to less-selected clinical populations is rarely tested.

As well, a limitation in the existing evidence base is the lack of means of collapsing risk factors to arrive at a single estimate of risk. That is, although numerous studies examine overlapping groups of risk factors, the clinician cannot draw strong conclusions about the relative importance of these risk factors, nor their utility in aggregate. The persistence of this problem may be driven by more general reluctance among investigators to develop predictive models rather than testing specific hypotheses in a traditional fashion.[11] The availability of large, well-characterized, but unselected clinical cohorts, as, for example, from electronic medical records or national registries, may help alleviate this shortcoming.

Another strategy for improving diagnosis, beyond the development of risk predictors, may be the greater use of standardized assessments. For example, multiple self-report measures that capture mixed or hypomanic features during depressive episodes have been developed.[52,53] Integrating such self-report measures with careful characterization of longitudinal course may provide the best cross-sectional strategy for diagnosis. Nonetheless, consistent with Kraepelin's observations, only longitudinal follow-up truly allows for reliable diagnosis when individuals present in a depressive episode, at least until much-heralded biomarkers emerge. For both clinicians and patients, a willingness to recognize that any initial diagnosis is provisional, subject to later re-examination, could help to diminish the rates and consequences of misdiagnosis of these 2 disorders.

ACKNOWLEDGMENTS

The authors wish to dedicate this article to 2 respected colleagues who made crucial contributions to the understanding of mood disorder nosology, Athanasios Koukopoulos and Franco Benazzi.

REFERENCES

1. Goodwin FK, Jamison KR. Manic-depressive illness: bipolar disorders and recurrent depression. 2nd edition. Oxford (United Kingdom): Oxford Ed; 2007.
2. American Psychiatric Association. DSM-5-Diagnostic and statistical manual of mental disorders. 5th edition. Washington, DC: American Psychiatric Association; 2013.
3. Ghaemi SN, Hsu DJ, Soldani F, et al. Antidepressants in bipolar disorder: the case for caution. Bipolar Disord 2003;5(6):421–33. Available at: http://www.ncbi.nlm.nih.gov/pubmed/14636365.
4. Ghaemi SN, Ostacher MM, El-Mallakh RS, et al. Antidepressant discontinuation in bipolar depression: a Systematic Treatment Enhancement Program for Bipolar Disorder (STEP-BD) randomized clinical trial of long-term effectiveness and safety. J Clin Psychiatry 2010;71(4):372–80.
5. Yatham LN, Vieta E, Goodwin GM, et al, Agomelatine Study Group. Agomelatine or placebo as adjunctive therapy to a mood stabiliser in bipolar I

depression: randomised double-blind placebo-controlled trial. Br J Psychiatry 2015. [Epub ahead of print].

6. Ghaemi SN, Vöhringer PA, Patkar A, et al. Citalopram for acute and preventive efficacy in bipolar depression (CAPE-BD): a double-blind randomized, placebo-controlled trial. Am J Psychiatry, in press.

7. McGirr A, Vöhringer PA, Ghaemi SN, et al. The safety and efficacy of adjunctive modern antidepressant therapy with a mood stabilizer or antipsychotic in acute bipolar depression: a meta-analysis of randomized placebo controlled trials. Am J Psychiatry, in press.

8. Rush AJ, Trivedi MH, Wisniewski SR, et al. Acute and longer-term outcomes in depressed outpatients requiring one or several treatment steps: a STAR*D report. Am J Psychiatry 2006;163(11):1905–17.

9. Kirsch I, Deacon BJ, Huedo-Medina TB, et al. Initial severity and antidepressant benefits: a meta-analysis of data submitted to the Food and Drug Administration. PLoS Med 2008;5(2):e45.

10. Vohringer PA, Ghaemi SN. Solving the antidepressant efficacy question: effect sizes in major depressive disorder. Clin Ther 2011;33(12):B49–61.

11. Perlis RH, Uher R, Ostacher M, et al. Association between bipolar spectrum features and treatment outcomes in outpatients with major depressive disorder. Arch Gen Psychiatry 2011;68(4):351–60.

12. Akiskal HS. Validating 'hard' and 'soft' phenotypes within the bipolar spectrum: continuity or discontinuity? J Affect Disord 2003;73(1–2):1–5. Available at: http://www.ncbi.nlm.nih.gov/pubmed/12507732.

13. Sachs GS, Nierenberg AA, Calabrese JR, et al. Effectiveness of adjunctive antidepressant treatment for bipolar depression. N Engl J Med 2007;356(17):1711–22.

14. Koukopoulos A, Sani G. DSM-5 criteria for depression with mixed features: a farewell to mixed depression. Acta Psychiatr Scand 2014;129(1):4–16.

15. Sani G, Napoletano F, Vohringer PA, et al. Mixed depression: clinical features and predictors of its onset associated with antidepressant use. Psychother Psychosom 2014;83(4):213–21.

16. Murray ML, Thompson M, Santosh PJ, et al. Effects of the Committee on Safety of Medicines advice on antidepressant prescribing to children and adolescents in the UK. Drug Saf 2005;28(12):1151–7. Available at: http://www.ncbi.nlm.nih.gov/pubmed/16329717.

17. van Praag HM. Why has the antidepressant era not shown a significant drop in suicide rates? Crisis 2002;23(2):77–82.

18. Perlis RH. Misdiagnosis of bipolar disorder. Am J Manag Care 2005;11(9 Suppl):S271–4. Available at: http://www.ncbi.nlm.nih.gov/pubmed/16232009.

19. Ruggero CJ, Zimmerman M, Chelminski I, et al. Borderline personality disorder and the misdiagnosis of bipolar disorder. J Psychiatr Res 2010;44(6):405–8.

20. Ghaemi SN, Ko JY, Goodwin FK. "Cade's disease" and beyond: misdiagnosis, antidepressant use, and a proposed definition for bipolar spectrum disorder. Can J Psychiatry 2002;47(2):125–34. Available at: http://www.ncbi.nlm.nih.gov/entrez/query.fcgi?cmd=Retrieve&db=PubMed&dopt=Citation&list_uids=11926074.

21. Benazzi F. Underdiagnosis of bipolar II disorders in the community. J Clin Psychiatry 2003;64(9):1130–1. Available at: http://www.ncbi.nlm.nih.gov/pubmed/14628991.

22. Smith DJ, Ghaemi N. Is underdiagnosis the main pitfall when diagnosing bipolar disorder? Yes. BMJ 2010;340:c854.

23. Berk M, Dodd S. Bipolar II disorder: a review. Bipolar Disord 2005;7(1):11–21.

24. Swartz HA, Frank E, Cheng Y. A randomized pilot study of psychotherapy and quetiapine for the acute treatment of bipolar II depression. Bipolar Disord 2012; 14(2):211–6.
25. Benazzi F, Akiskal HS. Refining the evaluation of bipolar II: beyond the strict SCID-CV guidelines for hypomania. J Affect Disord 2003;73(1–2):33–8. Available at: http://www.ncbi.nlm.nih.gov/pubmed/12507735.
26. Perlis RH, Miyahara S, Marangell LB, et al, STEP-BD Investigators. Long-term implications of early onset in bipolar disorder: data from the first 1000 participants in the systematic treatment enhancement program for bipolar disorder (STEP-BD). Biol Psychiatry 2004;55(9):875–81.
27. Gunderson JG, Weinberg I, Daversa MT, et al. Descriptive and longitudinal observations on the relationship of borderline personality disorder and bipolar disorder. Am J Psychiatry 2006;163(7):1173–8.
28. Berk M, Dodd S, Berk L. The management of bipolar disorder in primary care: a review of existing and emerging therapies. Psychiatry Clin Neurosci 2005;59(3): 229–39.
29. Pavlova B, Perlis RH, Alda M, et al. Lifetime prevalence of anxiety disorders in people with bipolar disorder: a systematic review and meta-analysis. Lancet Psychiatry 2015;2(8):710–7.
30. Barroilhet S, Vohringer PA, Ghaemi SN. Borderline versus bipolar: differences matter. Acta Psychiatr Scand 2013;128(5):385–6.
31. Trede K, Salvatore P, Baethge C, et al. Manic-depressive illness: evolution in Kraepelin's Textbook, 1883-1926. Harv Rev Psychiatry 2005;13(3):155–78.
32. Swann AC, Geller B, Post RM, et al. Practical clues to early recognition of bipolar disorder: a primary care approach. Prim Care Companion J Clin Psychiatry 2005; 7(1):15–21. Available at: http://www.ncbi.nlm.nih.gov/pubmed/15841189.
33. Angst J, Gamma A, Benazzi F, et al. Toward a re-definition of subthreshold bipolarity: epidemiology and proposed criteria for bipolar-II, minor bipolar disorders and hypomania. J Affect Disord 2003;73(1–2):133–46. Available at: http://www. ncbi.nlm.nih.gov/pubmed/12507746.
34. Benazzi F. Chronic atypical major depressive episode in private practice: unipolar and bipolar II. Acta Psychiatr Scand 1999;100(6):418–23. Available at: http:// www.ncbi.nlm.nih.gov/pubmed/10626919.
35. Hantouche EG, Akiskal HS. Bipolar II vs. unipolar depression: psychopathologic differentiation by dimensional measures. J Affect Disord 2005;84(2–3): 127–32.
36. Moreno C, Laje G, Blanco C, et al. National trends in the outpatient diagnosis and treatment of bipolar disorder in youth. Arch Gen Psychiatry 2007;64(9): 1032–9.
37. Perlis RH, Brown E, Baker RW, et al. Clinical features of bipolar depression versus major depressive disorder in large multicenter trials. Am J Psychiatry 2006; 163(2):225–31.
38. Kessler RC, Berglund P, Demler O, et al. Lifetime prevalence and age-of-onset distributions of DSM-IV disorders in the National Comorbidity Survey Replication. Arch Gen Psychiatry 2005;62(6):593–602.
39. Kessler RC, Berglund P, Demler O, et al, National Comorbidity Survey Replication. The epidemiology of major depressive disorder: results from the National Comorbidity Survey Replication (NCS-R). JAMA 2003;289(23):3095–105.
40. Merikangas KR, Jin R, He JP, et al. Prevalence and correlates of bipolar spectrum disorder in the world mental health survey initiative. Arch Gen Psychiatry 2011; 68(3):241–51.

41. Hendrick V, Altshuler LL, Gitlin MJ, et al. Gender and bipolar illness. J Clin Psychiatry 2000;61(5):393–6 [quiz: 397]. Available at: http://www.ncbi.nlm.nih.gov/pubmed/10847318.
42. Jones I, Craddock N. Bipolar disorder and childbirth: the importance of recognising risk. Br J Psychiatry 2005;186:453–4.
43. Mitchell PB, Frankland A, Hadzi-Pavlovic D, et al. Comparison of depressive episodes in bipolar disorder and in major depressive disorder within bipolar disorder pedigrees. Br J Psychiatry 2011;199(4):303–9.
44. Perlis RH, Smoller JW, Fava M, et al. The prevalence and clinical correlates of anger attacks during depressive episodes in bipolar disorder. J Affect Disord 2004;79(1–3):291–5.
45. Benazzi F. Bipolar II disorder and major depressive disorder: continuity or discontinuity? World J Biol Psychiatry 2003;4(4):166–71. Available at: http://www.ncbi.nlm.nih.gov/pubmed/14608587.
46. Perlis RH. The emerging genetics of bipolar disorder. In: Yildiz A, Ruiz P, editors. The bipolar book: history, neurobiology, and treatment. New York: Oxford University Press; 2015. p. 181–90.
47. Perlis RH. Translating biomarkers to clinical practice. Mol Psychiatry 2011;16(11):1076–87.
48. Chen JJ, Zhou CJ, Lui Z, et al. Divergent urinary metabolic phenotypes between major depressive disorder and bipolar disorder identified by a combined GC-MS and NMR spectroscopic metabonomic approach. J Proteome Res 2015;14(8):3382–9.
49. Munkholm K, Peijs L, Vinberg M, et al. A composite peripheral blood gene expression measure as a potential diagnostic biomarker in bipolar disorder. Transl Psychiatry 2015;4(5):614.
50. Wolfers T, Buitelaar JK, Beckmann CF, et al. From estimating activation locality to predicting disorder: a review of pattern recognition for neuroimaging-based psychiatric diagnostics. Neurosci Biobehav Rev 2015;57:328–49.
51. Goldberg JF, Harrow M. A 15-year prospective follow-up of bipolar affective disorders: comparisons with unipolar nonpsychotic depression. Bipolar Disord 2011;13(2):155–63.
52. Prieto ML, Youngstrom EA, Ozerdem A, et al. Different patterns of manic/hypomanic symptoms in depression: a pilot modification of the hypomania checklist-32 to assess mixed depression. J Affect Disord 2014;172C:355–60.
53. Zimmerman M, Chelminski I, Young D, et al. A clinically useful self-report measure of the DSM-5 mixed features specified of major depressive disorder. J Affect Disord 2014;168:357–62.

Treatment of Bipolar Depression

Evolving Recommendations

Robert M. Post, MD

KEYWORDS

- Lithium • Anticonvulsants • Atypical antipsychotics • Anxiety • Substance abuse
- Rapid cycling • Neurotrophic factors • Psychoeducation

KEY POINTS

- Depression is the most common and most difficult-to-treat phase of bipolar disorder, and it is associated with multiple psychiatric and medical comorbidities.
- Antidepressant augmentation of a mood stabilizer is no longer a first-line treatment recommendation and is replaced by selected atypical antipsychotics.
- The comorbidities of bipolar depression and goal of achieving and maintaining remission almost invariably require complex combination therapy.
- After the atypical antipsychotics, most of the potential treatments and augmentation strategies are off-label, so careful monitoring and evaluation of individual patients is essential.
- A greater number of depressive episodes is associated with more cognitive dysfunction, brain abnormalities, and treatment refractoriness, such that early and sustained pharmacoprophylaxis is the key to treatment success.

INTRODUCTION

Treatment of bipolar depression is a critical problem in psychiatry, as bipolar depression is responsible for enormous personal and occupational losses, psychiatric and medical comorbidities, cognitive dysfunction, and many years of lost life expectancy. Bipolar depression is the more difficult phase of bipolar disorder to treat, and patients undergoing naturalistic treatment are depressed 3 times more than they are manic.[1] Despite the high prevalence of bipolar depression and its severe consequences, there has been a many decades-long deficit in clinical treatment research and studies of the syndrome. Conventional treatment of bipolar depression toward the end of the twentieth century typically included antidepressant augmentation of mood stabilizers. However, the past decade has seen increasing evidence that this is not only a generally ineffective treatment approach,[2–4] but one that may be counterproductive. Given

Bipolar Collaborative Network, 5415 West Cedar Lane, Suite 201-B, Bethesda, MD 20814, USA
E-mail address: robert.post@speakeasy.net

Psychiatr Clin N Am 39 (2016) 11–33
http://dx.doi.org/10.1016/j.psc.2015.09.001
0193-953X/16/$ – see front matter © 2016 Elsevier Inc. All rights reserved.

psych.theclinics.com

this evidence and new information about the efficacy of several atypical antipsychotics in monotherapy or adjunctive therapy of bipolar depression, recommended treatment paradigms have evolved toward the use of mood stabilizers with atypical antipsychotics and away from the unimodal antidepressants for the treatment of bipolar depression.[5]

However, treatment choices and sequences are confounded by a variety of factors. None of the mood stabilizers (lithium carbamazepine, lamotrigine, and valproate) are well documented for their acute antidepressant effects and none of them are approved by the Food and Drug Administration (FDA) for this indication. However, they are typically involved in the long-term prophylaxis of bipolar disorder, and bipolar depression breaking through these agents alone and in combination during preventive treatment is quite common.

Given the occurrence of a breakthrough depression, the addition of an atypical antipsychotic has become a primary recommendation in most treatment guidelines. Nonetheless, the treatment options for an emergent bipolar depression in the absence of mood stabilizer treatment are poorly delineated by the literature, although monotherapy with atypical antipsychotics is the only FDA-approved approach. Despite the emerging evidence of the inadequacy of antidepressant augmentation of mood stabilizers for bipolar depression, the unimodal antidepressants are still one of the most widely used treatment strategies.[6]

We briefly review the evidence of the inadequacy of antidepressants and the potential liabilities of their first-line use in the treatment of bipolar depression. The usefulness of the mood stabilizers in the treatment of acute bipolar depression also is reviewed, as well the data of the atypical antipsychotics. A major focus of this article is on the prevention of recurrences of bipolar depression, which is a primary objective of long-term treatment. This discussion again raises clinical treatment dilemmas about decision making because of a paucity of treatment research.

Another confounding variable is the high incidence of psychiatric and medical comorbidities in bipolar disorder, and these, too, have been inadequately studied. In particular, anxiety disorder comorbidity and rapid cycling are predictors of a poor outcome in the treatment of bipolar disorder, as is childhood-onset disorder. The treatment algorithms for these common variations have not been determined. Likewise, alcohol and substance abuse are extraordinarily common in the context of bipolar disorder and treatment of these comorbidities specifically in patients with bipolar disorder has rarely been studied. Therefore, one must make indirect inferences from the literature on studies of treatments for the primary disorders of alcohol and substance abuse as they might best apply to those with bipolar disorders who have these comorbidities. Given the paucity of treatment information about the acute and preventive treatment of bipolar depression, the clinician is at an extreme disadvantage in arriving at appropriate treatment algorithms for achieving and maintaining remission.

There is wide agreement that remission is the goal of clinical therapeutics, as partial treatment with resulting residual depressive symptoms appears to be a predictor and precursor to relapse into a more full-blown episode. Here again the literature is substantial about achieving improvement and clinical response, but virtually absent as to what maneuvers might be most applicable for achieving and/or maintaining remission in bipolar depression. Although there are a multitude of secondary treatment options available to augment the mood stabilizers (MS) or atypical antipsychotics (AA), evidence for their efficacy in bipolar depression is scanty and indirect. Nonetheless, in an effort to achieve the goal of remission, it becomes necessary to use a variety of approaches that are not yet supported by randomized controlled clinical trials and other accepted classes of evidence-based medicine. Therefore, in this article, we attempt to grade (1) the quality and strength of evidence for many of the suggested treatments, (2) their safety/tolerability, and (3) their potential utility for patients with bipolar disorder.

We acknowledge that this subjective school-like grading system is not likely to be agreed on by many clinicians and investigators, but offer these grades as a preliminary basis for discussion, consideration, and further revision in the near future as more evidence becomes available. We hope that new research will in fact change the strength of evidence and sequencing for many of the recommendations noted in this article.

Given that many of the potential treatment options are off-label and are better studied in other illnesses, in some of the tables, we, as noted previously, grade (1) the strength of evidence of effectiveness in these other illnesses, (2) the general safety and tolerability of a drug, and then (3) try to integrate these assessments to give a preliminary utility rating for the practicality of using the drug specifically in patients with bipolar disorder. As there are many different systems for grading the evidence in the literature, we try to make these ratings easy for the clinician to intuitively understand by using standard grade school/report card ratings of A, B, C, and D.

For (1) the strength of the existing evidence, the grades are as follows:

A = substantial evidence from at least one controlled clinical trial
B = large amount of data from partially controlled and opened clinical case series
C = a modicum of clinical and case series data including case reports
D = theoretic approaches with as yet relatively little data support

For (2) tolerability/safety, the grading is as follows:

A = excellent acute and long-term safety and tolerability
B = good tolerability with relatively minor safety issues
C = some acute or long-term safety concerns with relatively common side effects or rare serious adverse effects
D = substantial reasons for concern

For (3) the utility in bipolar disorder, ratings are as follows:

A = good direct or indirect evidence of efficacy and good tolerability (use endorsed)
B = some minor concerns about likely efficacy or tolerability
C = may be an appropriate choice, but the risk-benefit ratio requires consideration and/or close observation
D = likely inappropriate option because serious doubts about efficacy or safety

MOVING AWAY FROM ANTIDEPRESSANT AUGMENTATION OF MOOD STABILIZERS AS FIRST-LINE TREATMENT

A large variety of antidepressant treatments are clearly first-line agents for acute and prophylactic treatment of unipolar depression. In fact, long-term prophylaxis with antidepressants after effective acute treatment in patients with several prior depressions is recommended by virtually every treatment guideline. However, this approach is underappreciated by the public and underused for recurrent unipolar major depression. There is little recognition that the statistical significance of antidepressant continuation in unipolar depression is of enormous magnitude[7] and there is an approximately 75% reduction in depressive occurrences in those who continue on active antidepressants compared with those who discontinue their effective antidepressant with placebo substitution.[8] In addition, virtually every antidepressant modality increases brain-derived neurotrophic factor (BDNF) and neurogenesis, and longer duration of antidepressant use compared with shorter duration use is associated with preservation of hippocampal volume with aging.

Yet the situation is quite different in the treatment of bipolar disorder. Although widely used,[6] antidepressant monotherapy is almost never formally recommended in the guidelines as appropriate for bipolar depression, although Amsterdam and Shults[9] suggested their potential utility for those with a bipolar II depression. Accumulating evidence now also indicates that antidepressants even as augmentation of MSs are generally ineffective and improvement does not exceed that of placebo. The meta-analysis of Sidor and MacQueen[2] comes to this conclusion and suggests at the same time that there is little evidence for antidepressant-induced increases in switches into mania. However, other data suggest that some specific antidepressants, particularly those with noradrenergic potency, may be associated with a greater likelihood of switching into mania then other agents such as selective serotonin reuptake inhibitors (SSRIs) or bupropion.[10,11] There are a variety of characteristics of bipolar depression that appear associated with an increased risk of switching into mania on antidepressants even when used as augmentation of MS, as outlined in **Table 1**.

In addition to these potential liabilities, there is also evidence that antidepressants can increase cycle acceleration and there is a modicum of uncontrolled data suggesting that antidepressant use could be associated with an ultimately poor treatment outcome. For example, Post and colleagues[3] reported that the number of prior antidepressant trials before patients entered a treatment network at average age 40 was associated with a poor response to long-term prospective naturalistic treatment. Others suggest especially poor response to antidepressants in those with mixed states.

The recent overview on the use of antidepressants in the treatment of bipolar depression from the International Society for Bipolar Disorders emphasizes these reservations.[21] Nonetheless, antidepressant use continues to be widespread. This is likely based on many different factors. The efficacy of the antidepressants, as noted previously, is well documented in unipolar depression, and there is a long tradition of use of these unimodal antidepressants in bipolar disorder, which has not yet been overruled by the appreciation of the new evidence and enlarging database. Another factor in this regard is that a small subgroup of approximately 15% of depressed patients who respond to antidepressant augmentation of a mood stabilizer for several months appear to continue to do well with continuation as opposed to discontinuation of antidepressants over the next year.[22–24] The experience of a small percentage of patients doing well with long-term antidepressant continuation and prophylaxis and having more relapses into depression with antidepressant discontinuation would appear to color the perception of response in general and to continue to

Table 1	
Risk factors for antidepressant-induced mania	
1. Younger age	Martin et al,[12] 2004
2. BPI more than BPII subtype	Altshuler et al,[13] 2006
3. Rapid cycling (>4 episodes) in past year	Post et al,[4] 2012
4. "Mixed depression" (ie, activated, speeded up, racing thoughts)	Frye et al,[14] 2009; Valenti et al,[15] 2011; Goldberg et al,[16] 2007
5. TCAs > 2nd Generation ADs	Gijsman et al,[17] 2004
6. NE active > 5HT or DA	Post et al,[10] 2006; Vieta et al,[18] 2002; Sachs et al,[19] 1994
7. Substance abuse history	Goldberg & Whiteside,[20] 2002

Abbreviations: 5HT, serotonin; ADs, antidepressants; BP, bipolar disorder; DA, dopamine; NE, norepinephrine; TCA, tricyclic antidepressant.
Data from Refs.[4,10,12–20]

exert considerable influence on clinical practice. At the same time randomized controlled data of Ghaemi and colleagues[25] indicate that if a patient has a rapid cycling course (4 or more episodes per year), then antidepressant continuation even after 8 weeks of apparent good responsivity is associated with a poor outcome. Surprisingly, this is revealed as an increased number of depressive relapses occurring over the subsequent year, suggestive of an increased rapidity of cycling of depressions but not manias.

CURRENT FIRST-LINE OPTIONS FOR TREATMENT OF BIPOLAR DEPRESSION

Given the sparse evidence for efficacy and the likelihood for some potential harm with the use of antidepressant augmentation, one must look to other alternatives. If we assume that a patient has had a previous mania (so as to make the bipolar diagnosis) and has been maintained on a mood stabilizer but still experienced a breakthrough depression, consensus is building that augmentation with an atypical antipsychotic agent is among the preferred choices. Three AAs are currently FDA approved for the treatment of bipolar depression. These include, in order of approval, the olanzapine-fluoxetine combination, quetiapine, and lurasidone, with the likelihood that cariprazine will soon join this list. See **Table 2** for the number needed to treat.

Many investigators and treatment guidelines place the use of the olanzapine-fluoxetine combination as a second-line option because of its potential for side effects, including weight gain and other aspects of the metabolic syndrome. Quetiapine is FDA approved both as monotherapy and as an adjunct to lithium or valproate for long-term prophylaxis. Recent data also indicate that monotherapy with quetiapine is more effective than placebo in long-term prophylaxis. Thus, quetiapine has the unique profile of being effective in both manic and depressive phases of acute and prophylactic treatment. In addition, quetiapine is FDA approved for augmentation of

---

Table 2
Efficacy of mood stabilizers and atypicals: number needed to treat

	Episodes	Prevention of: Mania	Depression
Mood stabilizers			
Lithium	7	8	49
Valproate	8	22	11
Lamotrigine	9	23	15
Atypical antipsychotics			
Olanzapine	3	5	12
Aripiprazole	6	6	64
Aripiprazole	10	13	44
Risperidone (LAI)	4	4	−26
Risperidone (LAI) + Li/VPA	5	7	16
Quetiapine	4	6	9
Quetiapine + Li/VPA	4	8	6
Ziprazidone + Li/VPA	8	10	56

Abbreviations: LAI, long acting injectable; Li, lithium; VPA, valproate.
From Ketter TA, Citrome L, Wang PW, et al. Treatments for bipolar disorder: can number needed to treat/harm help inform clinical decisions? Acta Psychiatr Scand 2011;123(3):175–89; with permission.

antidepressants in unipolar depression. It is noteworthy that aripiprazole shares this latter indication of augmentation of antidepressants in unipolar depression, but is not FDA approved for acute treatment of bipolar depression. In the negative studies of aripiprazole in bipolar depression, the dose was aggressively increased and this was associated with an approximately 50% dropout during the study, such that the initial indications of statistical significance over placebo were not maintained at the end of the trial.

The other FDA-approved treatment is lurasidone, which shows evidence of efficacy in the acute treatment of bipolar depression both in monotherapy and as an adjunct to treatment with lithium and valproate. In contrast to quetiapine, lurasidone is relatively weight neutral, less sedating, and not associated with other aspects of the metabolic syndrome, such as increases in blood glucose or cholesterol.

Quetiapine shows a rapid onset of antidepressant effects, achieving statistically significant improvement over placebo within the first week of treatment. Its mechanism of action of antidepressant effects is not clearly delineated but could include a variety of options. It has a major metabolite, norquetiapine, which is a 5HT2 antagonist and 5HT1A partial agonist. It is a moderately potent inhibitor of the reupdate of norepinephrine. It also is moderately potent as an inhibitor of muscarinic cholinergic receptors, which is of interest as it has recently demonstrated that intravenous scopolamine induces rapid onset of antidepressant effects in as little as 1 day. Effects of quetiapine on BDNF are also potentially involved in its antidepressant effects, as quetiapine increases BDNF in the hippocampus and prevents the decrements in BDNF following uncontrollable stressors. Both quetiapine and norquetiapine are weak inhibitors of dopamine D2 receptors. This appears associated with a low incidence of extrapyramidal side effects and accounts for the fact that higher doses of quetiapine (400–800 mg/day) are required for it effects in mania and schizophrenia.

The side-effect profile of quetiapine appears directly related to the potency of receptor binding. It is most potent in inhibiting histamine receptors, and sedation, accordingly, is its most prevalent side effect. Sedation is usually adapted to, but approximately 10% of patients drop out because of this side effect. Moderate potency in blocking muscarinic cholinergic receptors is associated with dry mouth and constipation. The drug also is an inhibitor of alpha 1 receptors and this might be associated with orthostatic hypotension and accompanying dizziness.

Lurasidone has a different receptor potency profile. Among its most potent effects is a blockade of serotonin 5HT7 receptors, which some have linked to antidepressant effects in animal models of depression. It also is a blocker of serotonin 5HT2 and dopamine D2 receptors. Lurasidone also increases BDNF and prevents stress-induced increases. What is more clear-cut is its lack of potency in binding to histamine and cholinergic receptors, which likely accounts for its relatively low potential for sedation and anticholinergic side effects.

Lurasidone is much better absorbed on a full stomach after dinner or after a 350-calorie snack with maximum peak blood levels or areas under the curve of the drug being twofold to threefold higher than those achieved on an empty stomach. It, as well as quetiapine and aripiprazole, is metabolized by hepatic CYP-450 3A4 enzymes and therefore subject to drug-drug interactions, particularly lower blood levels from combination with agents such as carbamazepine which induce 3A4.

Although cariprazine as of mid-2015 has not yet been FDA approved, placebo-controlled trials indicate that a dosage of 1.5 mg per day (but not lower or higher doses) achieved significant antidepressant effects over that of placebo in the acute treatment of bipolar depression. It is noteworthy that this drug is a dopamine D2 and D3 partial agonist, like that of that of aripiprazole, but cariprazine shows greater potency for D3 than D2 receptors. Three studies have also demonstrated its antimanic efficacy compared with placebo and there was one positive study as augmentation of antidepressants in unipolar depression. It would appear likely that this drug will soon have to be factored into the first-line treatment algorithm for bipolar depression along with quetiapine and lurasidone.

MOOD STABILIZERS IN THE PROPHYLACTIC TREATMENT OF BIPOLAR DEPRESSION
Lithium

Lithium is the treatment of choice for patients with classic presentations of bipolar 1 (BP-1) illness. This includes those with euphoric mania, clear-cut episodes with well intervals in between, no anxiety or substance abuse disorder comorbidity, and a positive family history of mood disorders in first-degree relatives. Data suggest that lithium is less effective in long-term prophylaxis in those with greater numbers of prior episodes or rapid cycling, as well as the sequence of episode pattern of Depression followed by Mania and then a well Interval (DMI) as opposed to the MDI pattern.[26,27]

A number of other factors make the choice of lithium particularly appealing for acute treatment and long-term prophylaxis of bipolar depression. Lithium has the best evidence for antisuicide effects in patients with the recurrent affective disorders and there are even multiple studies suggesting that higher, although still miniscule, concentrations of natural lithium in the water supply are associated with a lower rate of suicide in the general population. Lithium also has a variety of neurotrophic and neuroprotective effects. In humans, it increases hippocampal and cortical gray matter volume. In animals, it increases Bcl-2 at blood levels below clinically therapeutic. In a variety of animal models of neurodegenerative disorders, lithium decreases the size of the lesions involved. The models include middle cerebral artery ligation to produce stroke, Huntington chorea model, and those for AIDS and amyotrophic lateral sclerosis. Preliminary data from patients with affective disorders suggest that there is a decrease in medical comorbidity and an increase in longevity in patients who are maintained on long-term lithium compared with other agents. Similarly, there are very preliminary data indicating that those who renew their lithium prescriptions are less likely to have a diagnosis of dementia in old age.[28] Strikingly, in nonpsychiatric patients with the syndrome of mild cognitive impairment, maintenance treatment with lithium 150 mg per day compared with placebo resulted in less cognitive decline over the 1-year study.[29]

Carbamazepine

Interestingly, many of the predictors of relative good response to carbamazepine are the converse of those of lithium.[26,27,30] Those with a good response to carbamazepine include those with BP-II illness, continuous cycling, substance abuse and anxiety comorbidity, mood incongruent delusions, and a negative family history of mood disorders in first-degree relatives. There is some evidence for acute antidepressant effects of carbamazepine.[26,31] In rapid cyclers, a year on the combination of lithium plus carbamazepine was more effective than a year on either agent alone.[32] Moreover, the side effects of carbamazepine are prevented by lithium in the realm of benign suppression of the white count (because of opposite effects on colony-stimulating factor) and in the induction of hyponatremia (because of differing effects on vasopressin-like effects).

Lamotrigine

The clinical predictors of response to lamotrigine are less well elucidated, but include fewer number of prior depressive episodes, a personal history of anxiety disorders, and most interestingly, positive family history of anxiety disorders and substance abuse.[26,33,34] Controlled studies have indicated that the addition of lamotrigine to quetiapine,[35] valproate,[36] or lithium[37] has greater positive effects than the addition of placebo. Thus, lamotrigine, which is FDA approved only for the prevention of bipolar episodes, particularly depressions, can be used with lithium, and anticonvulsant valproate, and the atypical quetiapine, making it an important component of the treatment and prevention of bipolar depression.

Valproate

Valproate carries the reputation of being effective in those with noneuphoric mania (ie, those with anxious, irritable, pressured, or dysphoric mania), anxiety disorder comorbidity, and, as it is FDA approved for the prevention of migraine, it is an obvious choice for those with comorbid migraine attacks. In patients maintained on valproate and experiencing breakthrough episodes, the addition of lamotrigine was more effective than placebo.[36] In this case, one has to be particularly careful about the drug-drug interactions, as valproate essentially doubles blood levels of lamotrigine and increases the risk of serious rash.

If 2 of these MSs are used in combination in the long-term prophylaxis of bipolar disorder, it is still relatively common for a major depression to break through pharmacoprophylaxis. This is perhaps best revealed in the study of Calabrese and colleagues,[38] where only a quarter of the patients with rapid cycling bipolar disorder were able to be even acutely stabilized on the combination of lithium and valproate even in the short term. When responders were then randomized to either monotherapy, more than 60% of patients relapsed, indicating that extremely low numbers of patients will do well on monotherapy. However, in a subsequent study, investigators in this same group found that when patients were inadequately stabilized on the combination of lithium and valproate, the addition of lamotrigine was no more effective in achieving mood stabilization in the long term than the addition of placebo.[39]

SOME BUT NOT ALL ATYPICAL ANTIPSYCHOTICS ARE EFFECTIVE IN BIPOLAR DEPRESSION PREVENTION

All of the AAs show antimanic efficacy, and when they are used in conjunction with a mood stabilizer, appear to show greater antimanic efficacy than the addition of the placebo.[40] However, the converse is not the case, as there does not appear to be a class effect of AAs for acute treatment or prevention of bipolar depression. The addition of quetiapine clearly is effective in decreasing the recurrence of both manias and depressions in patients maintained on lithium or valproate. It also shows efficacy over placebo in monotherapy for preventing mood episodes.

However, olanzapine, aripiprazole, ziprasidone, and risperidone, which are FDA approved for bipolar prophylaxis, do not show an independent effect on depression prophylaxis, although they do decrease overall episode recurrence in comparison with placebo. Lurasidone is approved for the acute treatment of depression either in monotherapy or as an adjunct to lithium or valproate; it has not yet been studied in long-term prophylaxis of depression. In light of the less than satisfactory rates of response and remission, even on combinations of MSs, the addition of an atypical approved for acute bipolar depression (quetiapine or lurasidone, and to a lesser extent olanzapine/fluoxetine because of concerns about long-term tolerability) would appear to be an option high in the treatment algorithm of bipolar depression prevention as well as acute treatment (**Table 3**). For all of the reasons noted previously, lithium, which is underused in the United States compared with Europe, should

Table 3
Combinations more effective than monotherapy in prophylaxis of bipolar disorder

Lithium (Li) plus carbamazepine (CBZ)	Denicoff et al,[32] 1997
Li plus valproate (VPA)	Calabrese et al,[38] 2005 (adults)
	Geddes et al,[41] 2002
	Findling et al,[42] 2005 (children)
VPA plus lamotrigine (LTG)	Bowden,[36] 1998
Quetiapine plus LTG	Geddes et al,[35] 2015
Atypical antipsychotics (AA) as adjuncts to Li or VPA	Most AAs are approved by the Food and Drug Administration as adjuncts to Li or VPA

Data from Refs.[32,35,36,38,41,42]

almost always be considered in the treatment algorithm. In one recent randomized comparison of lithium with quetiapine, both drugs showed similar degrees of efficacy on most measures, but there was a higher dropout rate for side effects on quetiapine. However, in another randomized comparison, lithium was superior to quetiapine on virtually all end points.

ADJUNCTIVE OFF-LABEL TREATMENT APPROACHES FOR BIPOLAR DEPRESSION

A variety of alternative adjunctive approaches are of the potential utility in the acute treatment of bipolar depression, but only a few have strong placebo-controlled clinical trial data to support their utility (**Table 4**). One of these is N-acetylcysteine (NAC), which Berk and associates[43] showed was more effective than placebo in reducing depression and anxiety, particularly after 8 weeks of treatment. NAC also has the advantage of being effective in many of the psychiatric and medical comorbidities that occur in patients with bipolar illness, including obsessive-compulsive disorder and substance abuse with many drugs, including alcohol, cocaine, marijuana, and nicotine.[44] Typical doses in most studies are in NAC 500-mg capsules, 1 twice a day for 1 week and then 2 capsules twice a day thereafter. As indicated in **Table 2**, NAC receives an A grade in each category for evidence, tolerability, and potential utility in bipolar disorder (**Box 1**).

The data supporting the use of vitamin D3 is much more skimpy, circumstantial, and indirect; 1500 IU is more effective than placebo in augmentation of antidepressants in unipolar disorder. In addition, a high percentage of patients with bipolar disorder, including children with serious psychiatric illnesses, show vitamin D3 levels below borderline or even outright deficiency. For these reasons and an A for safety, vitamin D3 is given an A for utility.

Folic acid is in a similar category as vitamin D3; however, it has consistently shown efficacy in augmentation of antidepressants in unipolar disorder in multiple placebo-controlled studies primarily in Europe. There is also one very small placebo-controlled study by Coppen and colleagues[45] indicating that folate may potentiate the long-term prophylactic effects of lithium. Data support the use of L-methylfolate 15 mg per day as an adjunct to antidepressants in unipolar patients. L-methylfolate would appear to be important for the some 15% to 25% of patients who show 1 of 2 common genetic variants resulting in deficient activity of the enzyme methyl-tetra-hydro-folate-reductase (MTHFR). These individuals would appear to require and benefit from L-methylfolate to a greater degree than regular folate. Because folate and L-methylfolate compete for the same transporter, those on L-methylfolate should not receive supplemental folate.

Table 4
Potential adjunctive agents for enhancement of effects in bipolar depression: subjective ratings of (1) strength of evidence, (2) safety/tolerability, and (3) utility for bipolar disorder

Potential Adjunctive Approaches to Bipolar Depression

	FDA Approved	I. Strength of Evidence		II. Safety/ Tolerability	III. Utility for BP	Comments
		BP	UP			
Lurasidone	Yes	+++	–	A	A	Metabolic neutrality
Olanzapine	Yes	+	–	B–	C	↑↑ weight and metabolic syndrome (mts)
Quetiapine	Yes	+++	+++Adj.	B+	A–	Sedation +↑ weight and mts
Aripiprazole	–	+/–	+++Adj.	B+	B+	Akathisia
Lamotrigine	–	+–––	–	A–	A	Slow titration to ↓ serious rash
Lithium	–	++	++	B+	A+	↓ suicide, ↓ dementia, ↑ telomeres
Ketamine	–	+++	+++	B	C	Effects in 2 h but lasts only 3–5 d
N-acetylcysteine	–	++	+	A	A	↑mood, ↓ multiple addictions
T_3	–	(+)	++	A	A	Effective with normal thyroid level
T_4	–	(++)	–	B–	B	Mild hyperthyroidism induced
Armodafinil	–	+/––	–	A–	B–	? Efficacy
Modafinil	–	+	(+)	A–	A–	Expensive, help fatigue and attention-deficit/hyperactivity disorder
Vitamin D_3	–	–	++	A	A	Multiple rationales for use
Pramipexole	–	++	–	B+	B+	↓BP, nausea, disinhibition
Agomelatine	–	(+)	+++	C+	B	Improves sleep, circadian rhythms in UP
Minocycline	–	(+/–)	–	B	C	Rare lupU-like rxn; anti-inflammatory/neuroprotective
Folate	–	+	+++	A	A	Vitamin B-9; decreases homocysteine
L-methylfolate	–	–	+	A	A	7 times better bioavailability than folate
Omega-3 fatty acids	–	(+/–)	++	A	A–	1–2.6 g DHA + EPA
Methylene blue	–	+	–	B	B–	Blue urine color
Pioglitazone	–	+	–	C	B	Risk of bladder cancer

Abbreviations: +, some evidence; ++, substantial evidence; +++, strong evidence placebo-controlled; +/–, equivocal; ?, questionable; ↑, increased; ↓, decreased; Adj, adjunctive; BP, bipolar disorder; DHA, docosahexaenoic acid; EPA, eicosapentaenoic acid; FDA, Food and Drug Administration; mts, metabolic syndrome; rxn, reaction; UP, unipolar depression.

Box 1
Spectrum of efficacy of N-acetylcysteine (NAC) in psychiatric syndromes, addictions, and other pathologic habits: placebo-controlled studies

I. Efficacy in bipolar and unipolar depression

II. Efficacy in primary illness that are often comorbidities in bipolar disorder
   A. Addictions: cocaine, heroin, alcohol, marijuana, nicotine, gambling
   B. Other: trichotillomania, obsessive compulsive disorder (as adjunct to selective serotonin reuptake inhibitors), autism (stereotypy and irritability)

Typical doses versus placebo: titration of dose of NAC to 500-mg capsules, 1 twice a day for 1 week, then 2 capsules twice a day.
NAC is available without a prescription from many health food stores.
Data from Post RM, Kalivas P. Bipolar disorder and substance misuse: pathological and therapeutic implications of their comorbidity and cross-sensitisation. Br J Psychiatry 2013;202(3):172–6.

Thyroid augmentation with tri-iodothyronine (T3) 25 to 50 µg has positive support in meta-analysis in the treatment of unipolar depression and only relatively sparse data suggest that it is also an effective adjunct in bipolar depression or ultrarapid cycling. It is noteworthy that T3 augmentation is effective in those with normal thyroid function at baseline.

There are several small open-case series and 1 adequate placebo-controlled trial of supra-physiological doses of levothyroxine (T4) increased by 100 µg per week to a final dosage of 300 µg per day showing greater efficacy only in women with treatment-refractory depression with bipolar disorder compared with placebo. A similar degree of improvement on T4 was also seen in male patients with bipolar disorder but was not statistically significant, as the placebo arm showed substantial improvement as well.

Augmentation of antidepressants with lithium in the treatment of patients with unipolar depression is supported by multiple placebo-controlled studies and would appear to be a rational augmentation strategy to use in virtually any patient with bipolar depression who is not already on lithium, especially in light of the multiple potential other positive properties of lithium noted previously. A number of other potential useful augmentation treatments are outlined in **Table 2**. One of the more interesting ones that deserves further study is the anti-inflammatory, neuroprotective, antibiotic minocycline at a dosage of 100 mg twice a day. Open data suggest that it may have some antidepressant efficacy in bipolar depression. What makes it particularly intriguing is that approximately one-third of patients with bipolar depression have some evidence of inflammation, as marked by increases in C reactive protein, interleukin one (IL-1), IL-6, or tumor necrosis factor alpha. In unipolar patients, the addition of cyclo-oxygenase 2 inhibitors (such as celecoxib) has shown evidence for greater efficacy over placebo, but the targeted use of these agents specifically in patients with evidence of inflammation has not yet been delineated. Whether minocycline would be more or less effective in bipolar depression in the context of positive inflammatory markers also remains for further study.

A very substantial controlled clinical trials literature supports the observations of acute onset (within 2 hours) of antidepressant effects in depressed patients (including bipolar) receiving intravenous ketamine (0.5 mg/kg infused over 40 minutes).[46] Effects typically last only 3 to 5 days, but given the associated antisuicidal effects, such treatment deserves consideration in suicide emergency situations, such as those frequently seen in emergency rooms. Attempts to extend the effects are just beginning to be pursued.

Intravenous scopolamine also has a rapid-onset antidepressant effect, and oral augmentation with scopolamine showed greater benefit than placebo in patients with unipolar depression.

One night of sleep deprivation also can have dramatic, overnight antidepressant effects that can be sustained by lithium cotreatment, phase advance, and bright light therapy. Somatic physiologic treatments of repeated transcranial magnetic stimulation (rTMS) and electroconvulsive therapy (ECT) remain important options for the incomplete or nonresponsive patient to pharmacotherapy. Both suffer from a lack of a systematic literature guiding continuation treatment after a good acute response. One study did find that right unilateral brief-pulse ECT was more effective than pharmacotherapy in continuation[47]. Transcranial direct current stimulation (tDCS) and use of rapidly fluxing low-level magnetic fields remain promising but inadequately studied approaches. Vagal nerve stimulation (VNS) is the only treatment that shows increases in responsivity with more chronic treatment and deserves further study. A recent 5-year follow-up registry showed superior effects of VNS compared with treatment as usual in both response and remission rates, as well as length of remission.

TREATMENT OF SPECIAL POPULATIONS
Ultra Rapid and Ultradian Cycling

In general, those with rapid or faster cycling frequencies are more difficult to treat and less responsive to most drugs and naturalistic treatment in general. One approach that deserves further research is that of the dihydropyridine calcium channel blocker nimodipine. The gene encoding for the alpha-1 subunit of the dihydropyridine L-type calcium channel (CACNA1C) has been repeatedly found to represent a vulnerability factor for bipolar disorder in genome-wide association studies. Convergently, the dihydropyridine calcium channel blocker nimodipine has some evidence of antimanic and antidepressant effects, particularly in patients with bipolar disorder with ultra rapid and ultradian cycling.[26] Choudhry and colleagues[48] randomized approximately 50 patients with bipolar disorder to 1 of 4 groups. There was an approximately 50% response rate in the lithium-alone group, whereas the combination of lithium and nimodipine resulted in a significantly increased (73%) response rate. With nimodipine combined with valproate or carbamazepine in the 2 other groups, the response rate remained in the range of 50%, suggesting the overall superiority of the lithium-nimodipine combination. Another retrospective study reported that a year on the combination of lithium and nimodipine was more effective than a year on either agent alone. Together, the randomized open data and the small placebo-controlled trial of nimodipine using an off-on-off-on design showing unequivocal efficacy of nimodipine, make the rationale compelling for further study of this drug both in the general population of patients who are bipolar depressed and especially in the context of those with the vulnerability gene CACNA1C.

Also suggesting the importance of this kind of study are the data that the CACNA1C gene variant is associated with early-onset bipolar disorder in the latest studies from the Mayo Clinic. Moreover, Davanzo and colleagues[49] showed that nimodipine yielded a long-term remission in a teenager with ultradian cycling between severe mania and severe depression when multiple other conventional agents alone or in combination were ineffective. A final rationale for the study of nimodipine are the data indicating that the blood elements of patients with bipolar disorder consistently show increased levels of intracellular calcium. The assessment of whether or not nimodipine is more effective in those with elevated intracellular calcium levels and/or the CACNA1C gene would have merit. In patients who are unable to tolerate effective doses of lithium, augmentation with nimodipine might be considered, as it has an absence of the common side effects of lithium, such as tremor, diarrhea, or weight gain.

Anxiety Disorder Comorbidity

There is a 30% to 50% incidence of an anxiety disorder comorbidity in patients with bipolar disorder, and when this is present, multiple studies have shown that it is associated with a relatively poor prognosis. Yet the treatment of anxiety disorder comorbidity in the context of bipolar illness has rarely been specifically studied (**Table 5**).

Therefore, the potential agents for the treatment of comorbid anxiety disorder listed are all based on indirect and inferential data. Surprisingly, a modicum of data suggest that the unimodal antidepressants, which one would think would be effective for anxiety comorbidity, do not appear to be very effective in patients with bipolar disorder and may even in some instances be counterproductive. In our international network, we found a low long-term response when antidepressants were used in the context of a wide range of other treatment options for patients with bipolar disorders, but those who had a comorbid anxiety disorders did especially poorly with antidepressants, being involved in a good long-term response only 18% of the time they were used (Post and colleagues, unpublished data, 2015). Thus, we give anticonvulsant MSs and atypicals with efficacy in bipolar depression much higher grades for those with anxiety disorder comorbidity than the antidepressants.

Gabapentin is of particular interest in the treatment of anxiety disorder comorbidities in bipolar disorder even though it is unequivocally not effective in the treatment of acute mania. Yet gabapentin has shown efficacy in a variety of anxiety disorders, including social phobia, and in one placebo-controlled study of Vieta and colleagues[11] showed efficacy in augmentation of previously inadequate treatments in patients with bipolar disorder, although not specifically in those with anxiety disorders. Most of the mood-stabilizing anticonvulsants (lamotrigine, carbamazepine, and valproate) have some effectiveness in anxiety syndromes, and perhaps these, along with the AAs, as noted previously, should be given greater consideration in the treatment of anxiety disorders and mixed depressive presentations in patients with bipolar disorder. NAC is again a very good augmenting option, as it improved anxiety in patients with bipolar

Table 5
Possible approaches to anxiety disorder comorbidities in bipolar disorder

Social Phobia	Panic/Agarophobia	PTSD	OCD
Gabapentin (A,A,A)	Gabapentin (A,A,A)	SSRIs (A, A, B−)	SSRIs (A, A, B)
Clonazepam (A, A, A)	Clonazepam (A,A,A)	Topiramate (C,B,A−)	Atypicals (A, B, A)
Antidepressants (A,B,B)	Antidepressants (A,B,B)	Lamotrigine (B, B, A)	N-acetylcysteine (A,A,A)
—	Valproate (B,B,B+)	Carbamazepine(C,C,B)	Topiramate (A, B, B)
—	Carbamazepine (C,E,B)	Atypical antipsychotic (A,B,A)	Lamotrigine (D, B, B)
—	Lamotrigine (B,B,A)	Benzodiazepines (D,D,D)	Carbamazepine (D,B,B)
—	—	Prazosin (A, B, B)	Gabapentin (D, B, B)

I level of evidence in primary disorder = first letter; II safety/tolerability = second letter; III utility in bipolar = third letter.

Abbreviations: OCD, obsessive-compulsive disorder; PTSD, posttraumatic stress disorder; SSRI, selective serotonin reuptake inhibitor.

disorder,[43] augmented the effects of SSRIs in obsessive-compulsive disorder, and is effective in trichotillomania.

Substance Abuse Comorbidity

Patients with bipolar disorder experience a high incidence (in the realm of 30%–50%) of abuse or addiction to alcohol or other substances of abuse. There are variety of treatments for patients with alcohol or cocaine abuse as primary conditions, but again these drugs have rarely been studied specifically in patients with bipolar disorder.[26] Thus, the drugs outlined and rated in **Table 6** are off label and require quite indirect inferences about their potential utility in patients with bipolar disorder.

The potential treatments of cocaine abuse disorders in patients with bipolar disorders are a particularly interesting example of some drugs that are highly likely to be effective in patients with bipolar disorder and others that it might be best to avoid. NAC, topiramate, and modafinil, all have positive placebo-controlled data in patients with a primary cocaine abuse disorder. Each has also been relatively well studied in patients with bipolar illness, and in the instance of NAC and modafinil, positive effects on mood have also been demonstrated in placebo-controlled studies in patients with bipolar disorder, making them attractive options. In contrast, the GABA-B agonist baclofen has positive placebo-controlled data in primary cocaine abuse, but it receives a grade of D for potential utility in patients with bipolar disorder because a previous double-blind study in patients with affective disorders had shown that it exacerbated depression.[26]

Despite these caveats, specific treatment of comorbid substance use even with un-approved agents is of great importance from multiple perspectives. A substance abuse comorbidity complicates treatment and provides a second difficult-to-treat chronic relapsing illness on top of bipolar disorder itself. Moreover, with repeated bouts of stimulant abuse, pathologic effects (such as dysphoria and paranoia) increase (ie, show sensitization rather than tolerance) and also show cross-sensitization to stressors and vulnerability to episode recurrence, yielding a positive feedback cycle propelling a progressive increase in illness severity and deteriora-tion.[44] In addition, many of the neurobiological effects of repeated stressors or bouts of substance use mirror or add to those already involved in bipolar illness, further exacerbating somatic and neurologic pathology.[50] These data and concepts also speak to the importance of education and attempt at primary prevention of substance abuse in adolescents with bipolar disorder who are at an almost sevenfold increased risk of becoming exposed and addicted compared with nonbipolar adolescents.[51] Women with bipolar disorder are at greatly increased risk for alcohol abuse compared with those in the general population, and prior difficulties with depression and anxiety are associated with this use of alcohol. Patients with bipolar disorder and comorbid substance abuse are at particularly high risk for marital, employment, and legal diffi-culties, as well as incarceration, homelessness, and suicide, such that attempts at prevention and treatment even with off-label approaches are imperative.

Childhood-Onset Bipolar Depression

Childhood-onset bipolar and unipolar depression are increasingly common and based, in part, on a cohort effect where every generation since the early twentieth cen-tury has shown an increased incidence and earlier age of onset.[52] The treatment of bi-polar depression in children is more poorly defined than that of mania,[53–55] although use of antidepressants has revealed a high incidence of activation, if not outright switching into hypomania/mania. Open clinical studies have suggested the utility of lamotrigine in adolescents with bipolar depression. A recent placebo-controlled study

Table 6
Possible approaches to substance abuse comorbidity in bipolar illness

	I. Evidence in:		II. Tolerability	III. Likely Utility	Comment
	1°	BP			
Potential Approaches to Comorbid: Alcoholism					
N-acetylcysteine	A	0	A	A	Nonprescription
Gabapentin	A	0	A−	A	—
Topiramate	A	0	C	B+	Cognitive dysfunction, word finding difficulty
Zonisamide	A	0	B	B+	—
Naltrexone	A	(A)	A	B+	FDA approved for 1 alcoholics
Valproate	?	0	A−	A−	Nonprescription
Carbamazepine	B/C	0	B/C	B	Widely used in Europe long-term for anxiety and dysphoria
Acamprostate	A	(B)	B+	B−	FDA approved for primary alcoholics
Potential Approaches to Comorbid: Stimulant/Cocaine Addiction					
N-acetylcysteine	A	0	A	A	Available
Modafinil (Provigil)	A	0	A−	A−	↑Cost
Topiramate (Topamax)	A	0	C	B	Cognitive impairments
Disulfiram	A	0	C	C−	? Mood effects

Abbreviations: ↑, increased cost; ?, questionable mood effects; 1°, in primary alcoholism or stimulant abuse; BP, in patients with bipolar disorder; FDA, Food and Drug Administration.

demonstrated effective episode prevention of lamotrigine in child and adolescent bipolar disorder.[56]

rTMS also has been used successfully is small open studies of adolescents with acute depression. Interestingly, although immediate and extended release quetiapine has repeatedly been demonstrated to have efficacy in adults with bipolar depression, quetiapine XR failed to separate from placebo in adolescents with bipolar depression.[56]

A key unanswered question is, what is the best approach to a depression (in absence of a prior mania) in an at-risk child because of a positive family history of bipolar disorder? The literature remains mixed as to whether early use of antidepressants is associated with a subsequent increased risk for mania, and because unipolar depression is more common than bipolar depression, many investigators would still endorse the use of antidepressants for childhood-onset depression. Nevertheless, this should be done with caution, as childhood-onset depression is associated with an approximately 35% risk of a subsequent bipolar disorder diagnosis. Given the evidence for acute antidepressant effects of omega-3 fatty acids in adults, a modicum of data in children, and an excellent profile of safety, use of 1 to 2 g of the combination of docosahexaenoic acid (DHA) and eicosapentaenoic acid (EPA) would appear to have merit. Vitamin D3 augmentation, especially in those with low blood levels is also endorsed even in the absence of definitive data on efficacy. Further studies of presumptive unipolar depression in those with a positive family history of bipolar disorder and in children and adolescents with a bipolar depression is a pressing unmet need.

Such studies would be of great importance because, compared with adolescent and adult onsets, those with childhood onset of both unipolar and bipolar depressions carry a poorer long-term prognosis.[3,57] In addition, those with early-onset bipolar depression typically have a long delay to first treatment, and this delay in and of itself is associated with a more adverse course of illness, particularly greater severity and duration of depression in adulthood compared with those with adult onsets. Greater attention to childhood onsets of bipolar depression is indicated, given the association of an earlier age of onset of bipolar disorder with a greater degree of loading for multiple psychiatric illnesses in parents and grandparents of patients.[58] The total burden of childhood adversity is also significantly correlated with an earlier age of onset.[59]

One definitive recommendation is based on the studies for family-focused treatment (FFT) in those (with prodromal illness such as anxiety disorder, depression, or cyclothymia) with a positive family history of bipolar disorder.[60] These investigators found multiple measures of a positive outcome in those treated with FFT compared with treatment as usual. This was especially the case in families with high expressed emotion. Therefore, one must consider FFT or some related psychotherapeutic/educational intervention an ideal option for children with depressive and anxiety difficulties when there is also a positive family history of bipolar disorder. Offspring of a parent with bipolar disorder are at higher risk of a depression or anxiety disorder than even bipolar disorder, and 74% of the offspring will have a major psychiatric disorder on 6-year follow-up.[61]

Medical Comorbidities

Bipolar disorder carries among the highest burden of medical comorbidities among the psychiatric illnesses. Cardiovascular illness (myocardial infarction and stroke) is the major contributor to 1 to 2 decades of premature loss of life expectancy. Therefore, addressing the host of risk factors for cardiovascular disease (including obesity; smoking; lack of exercise; and high cholesterol, triglycerides, blood sugar, and blood pressure) would have particular merit. Statins for hyperlipidemia are import not only for their reductions in lipids, but suggestive data on depression preventive effects in women followed prospectively who were on statins compared with those who were not.

Weight gain can be approached with good diet and exercise supplemented by a number of promising medications. These include, in sequence of the magnitude of their effects, the combination of bupropion XR 150 to 300 mg and naltrexone 50 mg, often with an average loss of 10% of body fat; the anticonvulsants topiramate and zonisamide; and to a lesser extent metformin.

Active help with smoking cessation should also be pursued, as evidence suggests that patients are at higher risk for nicotine addiction than the general population, but have a similar quit rate. A host of other medical comorbidities in adults are related to the severity of adversities that patients experienced as children.[62] These includes asthma, migraine, menstrual irregularities, gastrointestinal upset, arthritis and autoimmune disease, head trauma, and the like. Each requires additional appropriate treatment and attempts at prevention, and whether psychotherapeutic intervention would help lower this medical burden or the associated more adverse course of bipolar disorder related to childhood stressors is not known.

Cognitive Dysfunction

One comorbidity of particular note is the development of cognitive dysfunction, present even during periods of euthymia, which occurs as a function of the number of previous episodes of depression and/or mania.[50] Principles of treatment of cognitive deficits thus include aggressive pharmacoprophylaxis particularly involving: lithium; dose reduction or elimination of sedating and impairing treatments; augmentation with bupropion or modafinil for their attention-promoting effects (before the use of stimulants); and, last, the cholinesterase inhibitors and/or memantine for outright dementia. Use of pramipexole and nutraceuticals, such as citicoline, have also received preliminary support.

SUMMARY OF PRINCIPLES OF COMPLEX COMBINATION THERAPY

Some general principles of therapeutics of this complicated, pleiotropic, and potentially recurrent and progressive disorder are listed in **Box 2**. Most fall under the rubric of early intervention and long-term prevention and continuous patient monitoring and education. Monitoring is critical for early intervention when hypomanic or mild depressive changes begin to appear, and prospective discussion of the symptom thresholds for added intervention should be discussed and agreed on with the patient. Careful monitoring is important in the assessment of what treatments and combinations are working well for an individual patient. This is of overriding importance, as even FDA-approved agents typically yield response rates of only 50% and remission rates are much lower. Assessment of the effectiveness (or not) of a given treatment regimen for a given individual trumps any general FDA approval or set treatment guidelines in arriving at best options. With appropriate treatment, the illness can often be ameliorated and held in remission to the point in which it no longer or only minimally interferes with the patient's life. Conversely, with casual or inadequate treatment, bipolar illness may run a progressively deteriorating course with devastating consequences.

The most compelling data for early aggressive, multimodal expert treatment are those of Kessing and colleagues[63] in patients hospitalized for a first mania and then followed for another 6 years. Randomization to a specialty clinic for only the first 2 years compared with treatment as usual resulted in many fewer hospitalizations, and greater compliance and satisfaction, not only during the 2 years of specialty treatment, but over the next 4 years as well.

Box 2
Principles of rational polypsychopharmacotherapy

- Add one major drug at a time (to evaluate effectiveness and side effects of new agent)
- Augmentation saves time over substitution (especially in the face of nonresponse)
- Consider predominant affective target (mania, depression, mixed state) and comorbidities in initial choice of a mood stabilizer
- Equally consider the long-term side-effects profile and overall tolerability of drug for its use in combination strategies in preparation for prophylactic use
- Add drugs with different mechanisms of action (and from different classes)
- Titrate a drug to optimal effectiveness and to a dose below its side-effects threshold (not to conventional dose/blood levels)
- Consider the presence of a positive family history of affective and anxiety disorders and family history of specific drug response
- Emphasize lithium and psychotherapy for management of suicidality
- Simplify dosage regimen to enhance compliance (ie, only bedtime or morning dosing, if possible), but achieving remission even with drug complexity fosters adherence
- Anticipate and manage predicted pharmacokinetic interactions
- In presence of side effects, decrease dosage of drug most likely implicated
- Follow emerging literature on clinical, neurochemical, and genetic predictors of individual response to individual agents
- Have patient (or a family member) daily chart medications, mood, sleep, comorbid symptoms, and side effects to help optimize pharmacotherapy; agree on early warning signs and symptoms of an impending episode and on appropriate action should they occur
- Such systematic monitoring will elucidate treatment response and nonresponse for that individual
- Monitor side effects (eg, cognition/sedation/unsteadiness) and comorbid conditions (alcohol and substance abuse and anxiety) as carefully as mood
- In the face of an excellent response, be conservative and maintain full-dose treatment into continuation and prophylaxis (in absence of side effects)
- In the absence of a good response, consider major changes in the core treatment strategies and then more unconventional and experimental approaches as required until effectiveness is achieved
- If there is a paucity of systematic clinical trial data (as is the case in bipolar disorder after first-line and second-line treatments), practice by traditional standards of "evidence-based medicine" will be untenable
- An individual's response and/or side effects trumps conventional Food and Drug Administration and treatment guidelines

As seen in this overview, the treatment of bipolar illness is an evolving art and science, made difficult by the paucity of treatment studies in children and adults. It is hoped that many of the preliminary recommendations outlined here will soon be either supported by new data or found wanting (**Box 3**). However, in one's own practice, matching the excellence of ongoing education, monitoring, pharmacotherapy, and psychotherapy of a specialty clinic[63] is a certain way to help patients better navigate the vicissitudes of bipolar depression.

Box 3
Possible treatment sequences for bipolar depression as a function of family history, presentation, and comorbidities

I. Family history: +BP/UP

A. Lithium (BP I/II)

B. For breakthrough depression: Add lamotrigine (LTG)

C. Adjuncts folate vitamin D_3 N-acetylcysteine (NAC) T3

D. If improvement stalls: Add memantine

E. For prominent anxiety/insomnia: Add quetiapine

F. If overweight/diabetic: add lurasidone

G. If still anxious add valproate + as needed gabapentin

H. If retarded: add bupropion H1

I. If still low and slow add modafinil armodafinil

J. Repeated transcranial magnetic stimulation; RUL (right unilateral) – electroconvulsive therapy

K. High-dose T4 mAOI (monoamine oxidase inhibitor)

II. Family history: no BP

A. Carbamazepine (CBZ)
   1. BP II++
   2. Anxiety and substance abuse ++
   3. Mood incongruent delusions ++
   4. Continuous cycling++
   A. *Then begin A. through L. (as above)*

III. Valproate (VPA) +/– Family history
   1. Dysphoric mania ++
   2. Anxiety ++
   3. Alcohol ++
   4. Migraine +++

Then to A. through L. (as above) (halve dose of LTG, as VPA doubles LTG blood levels)

IV. Family history: anxiety

A. LTG
   1. BP II++
   Then A. and then C. through J.
   2. Anxiety ++
   3. Continuous cycling ++
   Then add A. lithium and C. through L.

Consider targeting comorbidites with drugs before comorbidities

Topiramate: alcohol, cocaine, bulimia, anger attacks

Zonisamide: alcohol, bulimia

Modafinil: cocaine, attention-deficit/hyperactivity disorder

NAC: cocaine, alcohol, gambling, smoking, marijuana, and in obsessive compulsive disorder (plus serotonin reuptake inhibitor)

VPA: migraine, anxiety, alcohol

Gabapentin: anxiety, social phobia, alcohol

++, effective; +++, effective and FDA approved

REFERENCES

1. Kupka RW, Altshuler LL, Nolen WA, et al. Three times more days depressed than manic or hypomanic in both bipolar I and bipolar II disorder. Bipolar Disord 2007; 9(5):531–5.
2. Sidor MM, Macqueen GM. Antidepressants for the acute treatment of bipolar depression: a systematic review and meta-analysis. J Clin Psychiatry 2011; 72(2):156–67.
3. Post RM, Altshuler LL, Frye MA, et al. Complexity of pharmacologic treatment required for sustained improvement in outpatients with bipolar disorder. J Clin Psychiatry 2010;71(9):1176–86 [quiz: 1252–73].
4. Post RM, Leverich GS, Altshuler LL, et al. Relationship of prior antidepressant exposure to long-term prospective outcome in bipolar I disorder outpatients. J Clin Psychiatry 2012;73(7):924–30.
5. McElroy SL, Weisler RH, Chang W, et al. A double-blind, placebo-controlled study of quetiapine and paroxetine as monotherapy in adults with bipolar depression (EMBOLDEN II). J Clin Psychiatry 2010;71(2):163–74.
6. Baldessarini RJ, Leahy L, Arcona S, et al. Patterns of psychotropic drug prescription for U.S. patients with diagnoses of bipolar disorders. Psychiatr Serv 2007; 58(1):85–91.
7. Davis JM, Wang Z, Janicak PG. A quantitative analysis of clinical drug trials for the treatment of affective disorders. Psychopharmacol Bull 1993;29(2):175–81.
8. Geddes JR, Carney SM, Davies C, et al. Relapse prevention with antidepressant drug treatment in depressive disorders: a systematic review. Lancet 2003; 361(9358):653–61.
9. Amsterdam JD, Shults J. Efficacy and safety of long-term fluoxetine versus lithium monotherapy of bipolar II disorder: a randomized, double-blind, placebo-substitution study. Am J Psychiatry 2010;167(7):792–800.
10. Post RM, Altshuler LL, Leverich GS, et al. Mood switch in bipolar depression: comparison of adjunctive venlafaxine, bupropion and sertraline. Br J Psychiatry 2006;189:124–31.
11. Vieta E, Manuel Goikolea J, Martinez-Aran A, et al. A double-blind, randomized, placebo-controlled, prophylaxis study of adjunctive gabapentin for bipolar disorder. J Clin Psychiatry 2006;67(3):473–7.
12. Martin A, Young C, Leckman JF, et al. Age effects on antidepressant-induced manic conversion. Arch Pediatr Adolesc Med 2004;158(8):773–80.
13. Altshuler LL, Suppes T, Black DO, et al. Lower switch rate in depressed patients with bipolar II than bipolar I disorder treated adjunctively with second-generation antidepressants. Am J Psychiatry 2006;163(2):313–5.
14. Frye MA, Helleman G, McElroy SL, et al. Correlates of treatment-emergent mania associated with antidepressant treatment in bipolar depression. Am J Psychiatry 2009;166(2):164–72.
15. Valenti M, Pacchiarotti I, Rosa AR, et al. Bipolar mixed episodes and antidepressants: a cohort study of bipolar I disorder patients. Bipolar Disord 2011;13(2): 145–54.
16. Goldberg JF, Perlis RH, Ghaemi SN, et al. Adjunctive antidepressant use and symptomatic recovery among bipolar depressed patients with concomitant manic symptoms: findings from the STEP-BD. Am J Psychiatry 2007;164(9):1348–55.
17. Gijsman HJ, Geddes JR, Rendell JM, et al. Antidepressants for bipolar depression: a systematic review of randomized, controlled trials. Am J Psychiatry 2004;161(9):1537–47.

18. Vieta E, Martinez-Aran A, Goikolea JM, et al. A randomized trial comparing paroxetine and venlafaxine in the treatment of bipolar depressed patients taking mood stabilizers. J Clin Psychiatry 2002;63(6):508–12.
19. Sachs GS, Lafer B, Stoll AL, et al. A double-blind trial of bupropion versus desipramine for bipolar depression. J Clin Psychiatry 1994;55(9):391–3.
20. Goldberg JF, Whiteside JE. The association between substance abuse and antidepressant-induced mania in bipolar disorder: a preliminary study. J Clin Psychiatry 2002;63(9):791–5.
21. Pacchiarotti I, Bond DJ, Baldessarini RJ, et al. The International Society for Bipolar Disorders (ISBD) task force report on antidepressant use in bipolar disorders. Am J Psychiatry 2013;170(11):1249–62.
22. Altshuler L, Kiriakos L, Calcagno J, et al. The impact of antidepressant discontinuation versus antidepressant continuation on 1-year risk for relapse of bipolar depression: a retrospective chart review. J Clin Psychiatry 2001;62(8):612–6.
23. Altshuler L, Suppes T, Black D, et al. Impact of antidepressant discontinuation after acute bipolar depression remission on rates of depressive relapse at 1-year follow-up. Am J Psychiatry 2003;160(7):1252–62.
24. Joffe RT, MacQueen GM, Marriott M, et al. One-year outcome with antidepressant–treatment of bipolar depression. Acta Psychiatr Scand 2005;112(2):105–9.
25. Ghaemi SN, Ostacher MM, El-Mallakh RS, et al. Antidepressant discontinuation in bipolar depression: a Systematic Treatment Enhancement Program for Bipolar Disorder (STEP-BD) randomized clinical trial of long-term effectiveness and safety. J Clin Psychiatry 2010;71(4):372–80.
26. Post RM, Leverich GL. Treatment of bipolar illness: a casebook for clinicians and patients. New York: WW Norton and Company Inc; 2008. p. 1–666.
27. Post RM, Altshuler L. Mood disorders: treatment of bipolar disorders. In: Sadock BJ, Sadock VA, Ruiz P, editors. Comprehensive textbook of psychiatry. New York: Lipincott Williams and William; 2009. p. 1743–812.
28. Kessing LV, Sondergard L, Forman JL, et al. Lithium treatment and risk of dementia. Arch Gen Psychiatry 2008;65(11):1331–5.
29. Forlenza OV, Diniz BS, Radanovic M, et al. Disease-modifying properties of long-term lithium treatment for amnestic mild cognitive impairment: randomised controlled trial. Br J Psychiatry 2011;198(5):351–6.
30. Greil W, Kleindienst N, Erazo N, et al. Differential response to lithium and carbamazepine in the prophylaxis of bipolar disorder. J Clin Psychopharmacol 1998; 18(6):455–60.
31. Zhang ZJ, Kang WH, Tan QR, et al. Adjunctive herbal medicine with carbamazepine for bipolar disorders: a double-blind, randomized, placebo-controlled study. J Psychiatr Res 2007;41(3–4):360–9.
32. Denicoff KD, Smith-Jackson EE, Disney ER, et al. Comparative prophylactic efficacy of lithium, carbamazepine, and the combination in bipolar disorder. J Clin Psychiatry 1997;58(11):470–8.
33. Obrocea GV, Dunn RM, Frye MA, et al. Clinical predictors of response to lamotrigine and gabapentin monotherapy in refractory affective disorders. Biol Psychiatry 2002;51(3):253–60.
34. Alda M, Passmore MJ, Garnham J, et al. Clinical presentation of bipolar disorders responsive to lithium or lamotrigine. Int J Neuropsychopharmacol 2002; 5(Suppl 1):S58.
35. Geddes JR, Rendell J, Hinds C, et al. Comparative evaluation of quetiapine plus lamotigine versus quetiapine monotherapy in people with bipolar depression: a randomized trial (cequel). Toronto: ISBD; 2015.

36. Bowden CL. New concepts in mood stabilization: evidence for the effectiveness of valproate and lamotrigine. Neuropsychopharmacology 1998;19(3):194–9.
37. Van der Loos M, Mulder P, Hartong E, et al. Efficacy and safety of lamotrigine as add-on treatment to lithium in bipolar depression: a multicenter, double-blind, placebo-controlled trial. J Clin Psychiatry 2009;70:223–31.
38. Calabrese JR, Shelton MD, Rapport DJ, et al. A 20-month, double-blind, maintenance trial of lithium versus divalproex in rapid-cycling bipolar disorder. Am J Psychiatry 2005;162(11):2152–61.
39. Kemp DE, Gao K, Fein EB, et al. Lamotrigine as add-on treatment to lithium and divalproex: lessons learned from a double-blind, placebo-controlled trial in rapid-cycling bipolar disorder. Bipolar Disord 2012;14(7):780–9.
40. Ketter TA. Handbook of diagnosis and treatment bipolar disorder. Washington, DC: Am Psych Pub, Inc; 2010.
41. Geddes JR, Rendell JM, Goodwin GM. BALANCE: a large simple trial of maintenance treatment for bipolar disorder. World Psychiatry 2002;1(1):48–51.
42. Findling RL, McNamara NK, Youngstrom EA, et al. Double-blind 18-month trial of lithium versus divalproex maintenance treatment in pediatric bipolar disorder. J Am Acad Child Adolesc Psychiatry 2005;44(5):409–17.
43. Berk M, Copolov DL, Dean O, et al. N-acetyl cysteine for depressive symptoms in bipolar disorder–a double-blind randomized placebo-controlled trial. Biol Psychiatry 2008;64(6):468–75.
44. Post RM, Kalivas P. Bipolar disorder and substance misuse: pathological and therapeutic implications of their comorbidity and cross-sensitisation. Br J Psychiatry 2013;202(3):172–6.
45. Coppen A, Chaudhry S, Swade C. Folic acid enhances lithium prophylaxis. J Affect Disord 1986;10(1):9–13.
46. Zarate CA Jr, Singh JB, Carlson PJ, et al. A randomized trial of an N-methyl-D-aspartate antagonist in treatment-resistant major depression. Arch Gen Psychiatry 2006;63(8):856–64.
47. Schoeyen HK, Kessler U, Andreassen OA, et al. Treatment-resistant bipolar depression: a randomized controlled trial of electroconvulsive therapy versus algorithm-based pharmacological treatment. Am J Psychiatry 2015;172(1):41–51.
48. Chaudhry HR, Kahn RM, Shabbir A, et al. Nimodipine in the treatment of bipolar disorder. New Orleans (LA): Society of Biological Psychiatry; 2010. p. 232S.
49. Davanzo PA, Krah N, Kleiner J, et al. Nimodipine treatment of an adolescent with ultradian cycling bipolar affective illness. J Child Adolesc Psychopharmacol 1999;9(1):51–61.
50. Post RM, Fleming J, Kapczinski F. Neurobiological correlates of illness progression in the recurrent affective disorders. J Psychiatr Res 2012;46(5):561–73.
51. Wilens TE, Biederman J, Millstein RB, et al. Risk for substance use disorders in youths with child- and adolescent-onset bipolar disorder. J Am Acad Child Adolesc Psychiatry 1999;38(6):680–5.
52. Lange KJ, McInnis MG. Studies of anticipation in bipolar affective disorder. CNS Spectr 2002;7(3):196–202.
53. Geller B, Tillman R, Bolhofner K, et al. Pharmacological and non-drug treatment of child bipolar I disorder during prospective eight-year follow-up. Bipolar Disord 2010;12(2):164–71.
54. Geller B, Luby JL, Joshi P, et al. A randomized controlled trial of risperidone, lithium, or divalproex sodium for initial treatment of bipolar I disorder, manic or mixed phase, in children and adolescents. Arch Gen Psychiatry 2012;69(5):515–28.

55. Wagner KD, Kowatch RA, Emslie GJ, et al. A double-blind, randomized, placebo-controlled trial of oxcarbazepine in the treatment of bipolar disorder in children and adolescents. Am J Psychiatry 2006;163(7):1179–86.
56. Findling RL, Pathak S, Earley WR, et al. Efficacy and safety of extended-release quetiapine fumarate in youth with bipolar depression: an 8 week, double-blind, placebo-controlled trial. J Child Adolesc Psychopharmacol 2014;24(6):325–35.
57. Perlis RH, Miyahara S, Marangell LB, et al. Long-term implications of early onset in bipolar disorder: data from the first 1000 participants in the systematic treatment enhancement program for bipolar disorder (STEP-BD). Biol Psychiatry 2004;55(9):875–81.
58. Post RM, Altshuler L, Kupka R, et al. More pernicious course of bipolar disorder in the United States than in many European countries: implications for policy and treatment. J Affect Disord 2014;160:27–33.
59. Post RM, Altshuler L, Leverich G, et al. More stressors prior to and during the course of bipolar illness in patients from the United States compared with the Netherlands and Germany. Psychiatry Res 2013;210(3):880–6.
60. Miklowitz DJ, Schneck CD, Singh MK, et al. Early intervention for symptomatic youth at risk for bipolar disorder: a randomized trial of family-focused therapy. J Am Acad Child Adolesc Psychiatry 2013;52(2):121–31.
61. Axelson D, Goldstein B, Goldstein T, et al. Diagnostic precursors to bipolar disorder in offspring of parents with bipolar disorder: a longitudinal study. Am J Psychiatry 2015;172(7):638–46.
62. Post RM, Altshuler LL, Leverich GS, et al. Role of childhood adversity in the development of medical co-morbidities associated with bipolar disorder. J Affect Disord 2013;147(1–3):288–94.
63. Kessing LV, Hansen HV, Hvenegaard A, et al. Treatment in a specialised outpatient mood disorder clinic v. standard out-patient treatment in the early course of bipolar disorder: randomised clinical trial. Br J Psychiatry 2013;202(3):212–9.

Psychotherapeutic Treatment of Bipolar Depression

Kibby McMahon, BA[a], Nathaniel R. Herr, PhD[b],
Noga Zerubavel, PhD[c], Nicolas Hoertel, MD, MPH[d,e,f],
Andrada D. Neacsiu, PhD[c,*]

KEYWORDS

- Bipolar depression • Psychotherapy • Review • Clinical recommendations

KEY POINTS

- There are several evidence-based psychotherapy options for bipolar depression: cognitive-behavioral therapy, family focused therapy, interpersonal and social rhythms therapy, mindfulness-based cognitive therapy, and dialectical behavior therapy.
- There are promising additional psychotherapy options that are evidence-based for unipolar but need research for bipolar depression: behavioral activation, unified protocol, cognitive behavioral analysis system of psychotherapy, and others.
- Different psychotherapy approaches address different aspects of bipolar depression. Using evidence-based assessments, recommendations can be made for the most appropriate psychotherapy treatment of a particular patient.
- Psychotherapy for bipolar depression is intended as an adjunctive to medication management and should include several key elements, such as psychoeducation, increasing awareness of mood, establishing routines, and targeting medication adherence.

Disclosure statement: The authors have nothing to disclose.
[a] Cognitive-Behavioral Research and Treatment Program, Department of Psychology and Neuroscience, Duke University Medical Center, Duke University, 3026, 2213 Elba Street, Room 123, Durham, NC 27710, USA; [b] Department of Psychology, American University, 4400 Massachusetts Avenue Northwest, Washington, DC 20016, USA; [c] Cognitive-Behavioral Research and Treatment Program, Department of Psychiatry and Behavioral Science, Duke University Medical Center, 3026, 2213 Elba Street, Room 123, Durham, NC 27710, USA; [d] Department of Psychiatry, Corentin Celton Hospital, Assistance Publique-Hôpitaux de Paris (APHP), 4 parvis Corentin Celton, Issy-les-Moulineaux 92130, France; [e] INSERM UMR 894, Psychiatry and Neurosciences Center, 2 ter rue d'Alésia, Paris 75014, France; [f] PRES Sorbonne Paris Cité, Paris Descartes University, 12 Rue de l'École de Médecine, Paris 75006, France
* Corresponding author.
E-mail address: andrada.neacsiu@duke.edu

Psychiatr Clin N Am 39 (2016) 35–56
http://dx.doi.org/10.1016/j.psc.2015.09.005
0193-953X/16/$ – see front matter © 2016 Elsevier Inc. All rights reserved.
psych.theclinics.com

OVERVIEW

Bipolar disorder is a debilitating and costly condition,[1] and most of the treatment research has focused on the manic or hypomanic episodes that occur in the course of the disorder.[2,3] However, depressive episodes within bipolar disorder, referred to as *bipolar depression*, occur with higher frequency than manic/hypomanic episodes[4,5] and are also associated with premature death,[6] elevated risk for suicidal behaviors,[7] and significant functional impairment.[8,9] Thus, bipolar depression, independent from mania and hypomania, is an important target of intervention.

Although there have been impressive breakthroughs in the treatment of bipolar disorder with psychiatric medication,[10] none of the available mood-stabilizing drugs show sufficient efficacy in treating bipolar depression.[11–13] The response rate of patients with bipolar disorder to these drugs is only about 50%, even in patients with low psychiatric comorbidity rates.[14] Furthermore, mood stabilizers can potentially cause serious long-term health problems, such as the development of metabolic and cardiovascular diseases. Even for those for whom medication is successful, evidence has found a high rate of noncompliance with medication (up to 50%)[15] and an elevated frequency of residual depressive symptoms outside major mood episodes.[16,17] Taken together, these findings suggest that current treatments need improvement to better address bipolar depression.

In addition to mood stabilizers, adjunctive psychotherapy can greatly improve treatment outcomes.[18] Evidence has accumulated that brief, manualized psychotherapies are as efficacious as medication in reducing acute unipolar depression severity, have fewer side effects, and may be more efficacious in preventing relapse.[19,20] In this review, the authors present several psychotherapy options with direct evidence for bipolar depression as well as some promising avenues for intervention that are in need of research with bipolar disorder.

ASSESSMENT OF BIPOLAR DEPRESSION

Existing psychotherapies conceptualize bipolar depression as a collection of problems that can be addressed in therapy; therefore, detailed assessment of such problems is a necessary step in developing a treatment plan and evaluating progress. When a patient reports a history of depression (**Table 1**), history of manic or hypomanic behaviors should be assessed using the Structural Clinical Interview for DSM Disorders[21] or the Mood Disorder Questionnaire.[22] A bipolar disorder diagnosis should indicate that the provider should consider initiating medication (if not already administered), providing psychoeducation about the disorder, and targeting medication adherence.

Once providers have assessed (major) depression, it is recommended to examine whether patients ever had a background of manic or hypomanic episodes (as defined in the *Diagnostic and Statistical Manual of Mental Disorders* [Fifth Edition] [*DSM-5*]). Indicators that should make the provider particularly prudent and make him or her assess carefully for past history of hypomanic or manic episodes are

1. A family history of bipolar[23]
2. Atypical features, such as presence of hypersomnia[24,25] or leaden paralysis[26]
3. Psychosis[27]
4. Melancholic features[28,29]
5. Psychomotor disturbance[17,25,30]
6. Early age of onset, particularly before 21 years of age[31]
7. High frequency of episodes[25]

Table 1
Assessment tools for bipolar depression and associated problems

Problem	Assessment Type	Measures
Bipolar depression (presentation and severity)	Semistructured interview	• Structured Clinical Interview for *DSM-IV-TR* Patient Edition[21,126] • Schedules for Affective Disorders and Schizophrenia–Lifetime Version[127] • Hamilton Rating Scale for Depression[128]
	Self-report	• Beck Depression Inventory[129,130] • Patient Health Questionnaire-9[131,132] • Mania Rating Scale[133]
Dysfunctional cognition and behaviors	Self-report	• Automatic Thoughts Questionnaire[134] • Dysfunctional Attitudes Scale[135] • Beck Hopelessness Scale[136] • Ruminative Responses Scale[137]
Emotional expressivity	Semistructured interview	• Camberwell Family Interview[138]
	Behavioral assessment	• Category System for Partner Interaction[139] • Five-minute speech sample[140]
Interpersonal deficits	Self-report	• Social rhythm metric[141] • Social Adjustment Scale[142] • Inventory of interpersonal problems[143]
Suicidality	Semistructured interview	• The Suicide and Self-Injury Interview[84]
Comorbid anxiety	Semistructured interview	• Anxiety Disorders Interview Schedule[144]
	Self-report	• Beck Anxiety Inventory[145]
Emotion dysregulation	Self-report	• The Difficulties in Emotion Regulation Scale[146] (cutoff of 97 used to define high emotion dysregulation and enroll in DBT[87]) • The Avoidance and Action Questionnaire[147,148] • The Cognitive Emotion Regulation Questionnaire[149]
Mindfulness	Self-report	• Five Facet Mindfulness Questionnaire[150] • Mindful Awareness Attention Scale[151]

Abbreviation: DSM-IV-TR, Diagnostic and Statistical Manual of Mental Disorders (Fourth Edition, Text Revision).
  Data from Refs.[21,84,87,126–151]

8. Comorbid anxiety disorders, such as obsessive-compulsive[32] or panic disorder[33]
9. Presence of severe suicidal behavior[17,30]
10. Major depressive episode refractory to at least 2 lines of antidepressants[34]

After bipolar disorder has been diagnosed, it is also recommended that providers assess hallmark problems or complaints that increase the specificity of the clinical presentation. Within bipolar depression, psychotherapies have been designed to address problems, such as anhedonia and depressed mood, lack of motivation, suicidal behaviors, interpersonal difficulties, maladaptive thoughts, inconsistent routines, and difficulties managing emotions. Using evidence-based measures can help determine the presence and severity of such problems (see **Table 1**). Depending on which presenting problems are most severe, providers can recommend a psychotherapy protocol that meets the patients' particular needs. Effective psychotherapies for bipolar depression include cognitive-behavioral therapy (CBT), family focused therapy (FFT), and interpersonal and social rhythm therapy (IPSRT) or mindfulness-based treatments, such as dialectical behavioral therapy (DBT) and mindfulness-based cognitive therapy (MBCT). These psychotherapy modalities and their evidence are presented in the following sections. (**Fig. 1** contains a decision-making model of referring patients to an appropriate psychotherapy modality.)

COGNITIVE BEHAVIORAL THERAPIES

CBT[35] is a structured psychotherapy based on Beck's[36] cognitive theory that describes maladaptive thoughts and behavioral patterns that are instrumental for the development and maintenance of depression. CBT involves the use of several techniques, such as teaching patients to identify and modify maladaptive thoughts (eg, beliefs of worthlessness) or engaging in behavioral experiments to examine assumptions (eg, avoiding social interactions because of fear of rejection). CBT has been more recently adapted[37,38] to address thought and behavioral patterns specific to bipolar disorder.[39]

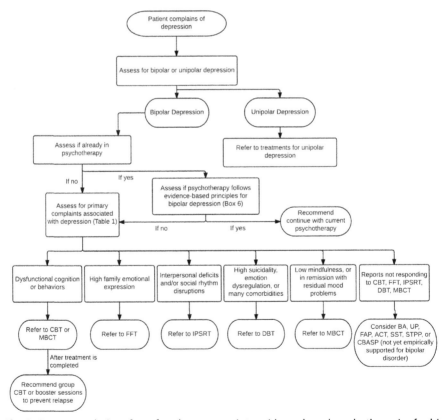

Fig. 1. Recommendations for referral to appropriate evidence-based psychotherapies for bipolar depression for medical providers. ACT, acceptance and commitment therapy; BA, behavioral activation; CBASP, cognitive behavioral analysis system of psychotherapy; DBT, dialectical behavior therapy; FAP, functional analytical psychotherapy; SST, self-systems therapy; STPP, short-term psychodynamic psychotherapy; UP, unified protocol.

Empirical evidence has demonstrated that CBT is effective in treating the bipolar depression.[40] In several randomized controlled trials (RCTs), CBT for bipolar (**Box 1**), administered by experienced clinicians, led to significantly higher reductions in depression severity and improvements in functioning as compared with a wait-list control[39] and to treatment as usual (TAU)[41,42] when controlling for baseline depression. Specifically, depression severity scores were cut in half over 20 sessions of CBT.[37] CBT may be less effective with patients with severe bipolar with numerous previous episodes.[43]

CBT was also examined during the Systematic Treatment Enhancement Program for Bipolar Disorder, a multi-site study that compared 30 sessions of intensive psychotherapy (including CBT) with a minimal psychosocial intervention in treating bipolar depression.[44] Compared with previous trials, this RCT had the most stringent control treatment, which included elements such as psychoeducation, relapse-prevention strategies, and illness management. Nonetheless, more patients recovered from their depressive episode within a year if they received intensive psychotherapy than the control treatment. Specifically, CBT significantly improved patients' relationship functioning and life satisfaction by teaching them to engage with others and challenge negative thoughts about relationships.[45] Taken together these findings support the efficacy of CBT for bipolar depression.

In addition to individual CBT, group CBT may also be effective in treating bipolar depression.[46–48] When compared with TAU, a 14-week CBT group treatment reduced depression severity significantly more and led to significantly higher improvements in social and emotional functioning.[47,48] Another clinical trial found only a trend in reduced depression severity after patients completed both phases of a 12-week CBT group treatment, with evidence that completing both phases was needed to improve social functioning.[46] These findings suggest that group CBT may be particularly useful to improve psychosocial functioning in patients with bipolar depression.

Box 1
Cognitive Behavioral Therapies for bipolar disorders

1. Theory: Depression is associated with maladaptive patterns of thought (eg, negative attitudes about the self) or behavior (eg, withdrawing from social contact). Thoughts, actions, and emotions all influence each other.

2. Goal: Patients and therapists agree on short- and long-term goals to address problem thinking or behaviors.

3. First phase: Psychoeducation about bipolar disorder and about the theoretic framework used in therapy is conducted.

4. Second phase: Patients and therapists work together on cognitive and behavioral coping skills that include
   a. Increasing awareness of cues that trigger mood shifts
   b. Cognitive restructuring to change negative thinking patterns
   c. Engaging in positive behaviors and within regular routines
   d. Keeping medication compliance high

5. Homework assignments encourage patients to practice skills in their daily lives.

6. Group CBT: Patients receive psychoeducation (phase 1) and practice skills (phase 2) in group settings.

Adapted from Basco MR, Rush AJ. Cognitive-behavioral therapy for bipolar disorder. New York: Guilford Press; 2005.

Both individual and group CBT show long-term maintenance of gains that are superior to control treatments for bipolar depression. Ball and colleagues[41] found that patients in the CBT group had a significantly longer remission than control patients. Lam and colleagues[49] also assessed the long-term effects of CBT on preventing relapse among patients with bipolar who were in remission. After 12 to 18 sessions and 2 boosters of a manualized CBT protocol, patients treated with CBT had fewer depression relapses and hospitalizations than did those treated with medication alone. However, CBT's effectiveness at preventing relapse was reduced at a 12-month follow-up and was no longer significant at the 18-month follow-up, even though coping strategies and social functioning continued to be improved.[50]

Although more longitudinal research is needed, the existing findings suggest that CBT (whether administered in individual or group format) is effective in treating and preventing relapse of bipolar depression; but the benefits are strongest during the course of treatment or shortly thereafter. Efficacy of CBT may be lower in patients with bipolar depression of high severity and with many past episodes of depression. These patients may, thus, need a more intensive level of care.

FAMILY FOCUSED THERAPY

Psychotherapy interventions targeted toward dysfunctional family interactions have also been found effective in treating bipolar depression. FFT was originally developed to target high expressed emotion (ie, critical, aggressive, or overly involved emotional expressions) in families of those who were at risk for schizophrenia.[51] Basic research has also associated bipolar disorder with high-expressed-emotion families and with maladaptive interpersonal interactions.[52] Thus, FFT was adapted and tested for bipolar disorder[53] (**Box 2**).

Several clinical trials have found that FFT effectively reduced bipolar depression.[54] Miklowitz and colleagues[55] compared 2-year outcomes of FFT and a crisis management intervention after acute mood episodes and found that FFT reduced depression severity significantly more than the control treatment. Improvements in family communication skills (especially nonverbal behaviors) were associated with improvements in

---

Box 2
Family Focused Therapy

1. Theory: Bipolar disorder is associated with high expressed emotion in families and maladaptive interpersonal interactions.

2. Goal: The goal is increasing positive interactions within a family and engaging the patients' support network in treatment and relapse prevention.

3. FFT protocol consists of 21 individual psychotherapy sessions conducted with the patients and their relevant family members.

4. First phase: Psychoeducation about bipolar disorder and the family communication style as a maintaining factor is conducted.

5. Second phase: Communication training is conducted (eg, learning and practicing effective communication skills, such as active listening or making eye contact).

6. Third phase: Problem solving is conducted (eg, assessing conflicts and developing solutions to address them).

Adapted from Miklowitz DJ, Goldstein MJ. Behavioral family treatment for patients with bipolar affective disorder. Behav Modif 1990;14:457–89.

bipolar depression.[56] FFT was as effective as CBT but more effective than a control intervention in leading to recovery from bipolar depression within 1 year.[45] In addition, FFT was also shown to be more effective in treating adolescent bipolar depression than a psychoeducational control group.[57] Participants in FFT had shorter depressive episodes, quicker recovery, and less depression severity over 2 years.

FFT may also have long-term relapse prevention effects. When compared with supportive individual therapy, FFT was equally effective in reducing bipolar depression during 1 year of active treatment. However, FFT prevented significantly more relapses than individual therapy within the year following the active treatment.[58] The investigators hypothesized that the long-term benefits of the therapy may be due to patients in FFT having the support of their family in monitoring mood and practicing coping skills. Therefore, FFT may be a preferred treatment of patients with bipolar depression who report family problems and poor social functioning, if their families are willing to be involved.

INTERPERSONAL AND SOCIAL RHYTHM THERAPY

IPSRT is a treatment developed specifically for bipolar disorder and consists of 2 primary components: social rhythm therapy (SRT) and interpersonal psychotherapy (IPT). SRT is rooted in research showing that disruptions of circadian rhythms, sleep-wake cycles, or social rhythms (ie, relationships or social demands that establish and maintain biological rhythms) may lead to subsequent affective episodes.[59] Although disruptions of biological rhythms tend to be more closely associated with the onset of manic episodes,[60] social rhythm disruption (eg, loss of a significant relationship or change in job) can be the precipitant of both manic and depressive episodes. Thus, the SRT aspect of IPSRT has the advantage of targeting both ends of the bipolar mood spectrum.

IPT is a well-established treatment of unipolar depression.[59,61] A systematic review[62] identified 13 outcome studies that evaluated the efficacy of IPT as compared with any other form of treatment, placebo, or a wait-list control. As compared with antidepressant medication, IPT had a similar rate of remission both acutely and during the maintenance phase. Combining medication with IPT led to higher acute remission rates than either treatment alone. Thus, IPT seems to be an efficacious treatment of unipolar depression, which led to its merging with SRT in the development of IPSRT to target depression among adults with bipolar disorder. IPSRT expands the IPT targets to include grief over the loss of the self: the person they could or would be if they did not have bipolar disorder. This additional element helps the client cope with any losses or changes in lifestyle and ambitions that come with accepting the limitations associated with the bipolar diagnosis. See **Box 3** for a description of IPSRT.

The largest study of IPSRT to date recruited 175 participants to receive IPSRT or intensive clinical management, a manualized medication management approach for bipolar disorder.[63] All participants were treated with lithium, augmented with antidepressant or antipsychotic medication when indicated. Results showed that participants in the IPSRT group remitted more quickly during the acute phase; among participants who remitted, those treated with IPSRT were less likely to experience an additional affective episode over the following 2 years. Most patients began the study in a depressed phase, and IPSRT was better than medication management at preventing a recurrence of either manic or depressive affective phases. Follow-up analyses indicated that improvement in social rhythm was a mechanism of change in IPSRT[63] and that participants in IPSRT showed better occupational improvement over the course of treatment.[64]

Box 3
Interpersonal Social Rhythm Therapy

1. Theory: Disruptions of circadian rhythms, the sleep-wake cycle, or social rhythms (ie, relationships or social demands that establish and maintain biological rhythms) lead to affective episodes. In addition, interpersonal problems are seen to be a maintaining factor for depression.

2. Goal: The goal is maintaining consistency in biological and social rhythms and improving interpersonal relationships.

3. IPSRT protocol consists of variable-length individual psychotherapy sessions targeting key elements:

a. Key SRT targets[66]
   i. Wake time
   ii. Time of first social interaction
   iii. Time of start of daily activities
   iv. Evening meal time
   v. Bedtime

a. Key IPT targets[61]
   i. Unresolved grief
   ii. Role transitions
   iii. Role disputes
   iv. Interpersonal deficits
   v. Grief over loss of the self

4. IPSRT treatment phases include the following[59]:

a. Initial phase (4–16 weeks):
   i. Psychoeducation about bipolar
   ii. Identify an interpersonal target
   iii. Orientation to social rhythm monitoring

b. Intermediate phase (3–12 months)
   i. Develop strategies and skills to maintain daily rhythms
   ii. Manage mood changes
   iii. Improve target interpersonal relationships

a. Preventative phase (2+ years, monthly)
   i. Maintain treatment gains
   ii. Prepare for potential future disruptions to social rhythms
   iii. Crisis management as needed

b. Termination phase
   i. Identify sources of support and resources available after therapy has ended
   ii. Prepare to tackle future difficulties without therapist

Data from Refs.[59,61,66]

More recently, Swartz and colleagues[65] have published promising pilot data indicating that IPSRT may be effective as a monotherapy for depressive episodes in bipolar II disorder. They report that 16 depressed patients with bipolar II who had been tapered off all medications had achieved remission after 12 to 20 weeks of IPSRT. Two additional studies found evidence that group ISPRT reduces depression severity in patients with bipolar disorder: one found this decrease after 16 group IPSRT sessions[66] and the other after 6 group IPSRT sessions in conjunction with 2 individual sessions and a telephone call at 12 weeks.[67] Miklowitz and colleagues[44] also demonstrated that patients treated with IPSRT recovered significantly faster from a depressive episode and were more likely to maintain remission than patients treated with just collaborative care. In summary, the existing data suggest that IPSRT is a promising treatment for reducing bipolar depression severity and preventing relapse in bipolar depression.

MINDFULNESS-BASED COGNITIVE THERAPY

Mindfulness-based cognitive therapy (MBCT[68]) is a group treatment protocol that uses a combination of meditation practices and CBT exercises to change the relationship that people have to their thoughts and emotions. This program, which is well established for treatment of unipolar depression,[68] has been successfully adapted for bipolar depression[69] (**Box 4**). The empirical literature evaluating MBCT demonstrates strong support for the reduction of depressive relapse, residual depression, and anxiety severity.[70–72] Some studies have shown positive results using standard MBCT for bipolar I and II disorders[73]; but most have modified MBCT in order to add attention to warning signs of anxiety and mania escalation, expanding the model that standard MBCT has for signs of depression and suicidal ideation.

Outcomes of MBCT for bipolar[69] investigations have shown that at the end of treatment, participants have a greater ability to observe thoughts and feelings in a less judgmental and reactive manner and experienced less depression.[73–75] In addition, they have greater concentration, less rumination, less emotional reactivity, and better cognitive and overall functioning.[76] These studies have had success reducing depression severity and relapse in remitted patients with bipolar disorder[73,75] as well as patients who are currently depressed.[74] One study compared MBCT for bipolar with TAU and showed significantly greater reduction in anxiety but not in depression severity.[77]

Experimental examinations using physiologic and functional MRI measures have shown that MBCT improves emotional processing,[78] attentional readiness,[79] emotion regulation, and mindfulness.[80] Taken together, these findings highlight that MBCT is most effective in treating cognitive and emotional processing problems associated with depression and can be used to reduce residual symptoms and relapse. Although

---

Box 4
Mindfulness-Based Cognitive Therapy for bipolar disorder

1. Theory: Automatic and maladaptive ways of thinking and engagement in contraproductive behaviors (eg, rumination, self-critical thinking, or avoidance behaviors) increase negative emotions and may lead to the development and maintenance of depression.

2. Goal: The goal is to increase early detection of depression relapse, change relationship to thoughts and feelings, and learn skills to change thinking and behavioral patterns that may lead to or maintain depression.

3. MBCT protocol consists of twelve 2-hour group therapy sessions in addition to biweekly individual sessions with patients where meditation and cognitive exercises are taught and practiced.
   a. CBT skills are taught, including behavioral activation and cognitive restructuring of maladaptive thoughts.
   b. Mindfulness component: In order to develop enhanced awareness, improve attentional control, and cultivate ability to detach from negative thoughts, patients engage in extensive meditation practice.

4. Beginning sessions: Recognize automatic pilot modes of thinking, feeling, and behaving and implement more effective strategies (cognitive-behavioral skills or mindfulness techniques) instead.

5. Middle sessions: Recognize warning signs of depression, anxiety, and mania escalation and cultivate self-compassion.

6. Later sessions: Develop an action plan to effectively respond to early warning signs of relapse into depression.

7. Homework: Homework includes 40 minutes of mindfulness practice daily and use of the CBT skills as needed.

Adapted from Deckersbach, T, Hölzel, B, Eisner, L, et al. Mindfulness-Based Cognitive Therapy for Bipolar Disorder. New York: Guilford Press; 2014.

patients experiencing a major depressive episode can benefit from MBCT, the research supports recommending this approach to patients with bipolar depression in full or partial remission who experience residual depression or anxiety.[70,74]

DIALECTICAL BEHAVIOR THERAPY

DBT[81,82] is a behavioral therapy developed originally for suicidal patients with borderline personality disorder (BPD). DBT (**Box 5**) is aimed toward patients who are multi-diagnostic, difficult to treat, suicidal, or who have difficulties managing emotions. DBT was developed using an emotion dysregulation conceptualization of BPD: those who meet the criteria for this disorder are thought to be more sensitive and more reactive to emotional cues as well as to have more difficulty returning to emotional baseline after an emotional response occurred. This biological vulnerability is worsened by insufficient learning in how to effectively regulate emotions and by overuse of maladaptive regulation strategies, such as suicidal behaviors, drug use, avoidance, or suppression.[81,83] DBT has been shown to be effective in reducing the use of maladaptive regulation strategies in BPD when compared with treatment by psychodynamic experts.[84]

Box 5
Dialectical Behavior Therapy

1. Theory: Heightened vulnerability to emotional cues coupled with lack of skills to effectively regulate emotions and overuse of maladaptive strategies to change emotions leads to pervasive emotion dysregulation that is common in BPD as well as several other mental health disorders.[85]

2. Goal: Increase understanding and awareness of emotions and improve emotion regulation and problem solving.

3. DBT protocol consists of weekly individual psychotherapy sessions focused on enhancing motivation and problem solving; weekly 2-hour group skills training sessions focused on teaching adaptive ways to regulate emotions, tolerate distress, be mindful, and address interpersonal problems; weekly consultation team for the therapist; and as needed phone coaching and crisis management to enhance use of skills in the natural environment. Typical duration is 6 months or 1 year. Adaptations of DBT have examined combinations of these 4 different components.
   a. DBT skills include mindfulness, emotion regulation, distress tolerance, and interpersonal effectiveness.
   b. Individual therapy is principle based and uses cognitive and behavioral techniques, such as behavioral and solution analyses, cognitive restructuring, and exposure strategies. It also includes DBT-unique strategies, such as dialectical, communication, commitment, and attachment strategies.
   c. DBT offers several evidence-based protocols to manage suicidality, therapy-interfering behaviors, calls outside of session, and case management.

4. Beginning 4 sessions include the following: Orientation and commitment to treatment targets, including addressing problems in a hierarchical fashion, prioritizing life-threatening behaviors, followed by therapy-interfering behaviors, and problems interfering with having improved quality of life.

5. Postorientation phase: Identify client goals and work through situational analyses to learn how to reach goals via use of skillful behavior.

6. Homework: Homework includes daily diary card tracking suicidality, goals, and use of skills.

Data from Refs.[81,82,85]

This conceptualization of BPD as an emotion regulation disorder can be extended to other disorders whereby problems managing emotions have been documented,[85] including unipolar depression.[86] There is mounting evidence that DBT adaptations are effective treatments for depression. For example, DBT skills training was significantly more effective than an active control group in reducing emotion dysregulation and increasing skill use in a transdiagnostic group of adults who met the criteria for anxiety or depressive disorders (excluding bipolar) and who reported difficulties with emotion regulation.[87] In addition, DBT components have been shown to successfully reduce (with large effect sizes) depression severity in treatment-resistant depressed adults[88,89] when compared with medication alone[88] or a wait-list control.[89] Depression severity also significantly decreased in an intensive outpatient program that included 5 weeks of daily DBT skills training and weekly individual therapy among multi-diagnostic patients (20% with bipolar disorder).[90]

Taking an emotion dysregulation conceptualization of pediatric bipolar disorder, Goldstein and colleagues[91,92] showed in a pilot open trial that DBT was feasible and acceptable and then in a follow-up RCT that DBT was successful in reducing suicidal behavior, emotion dysregulation, and depression severity in bipolar adolescents above and beyond TAU (differences correspond to moderate to large effect sizes). The treatment adapted standard DBT by including family members in the skills training groups (similar to other adolescent models[93]), offering fewer individual and group sessions, and providing bipolar-specific psychoeducation as part of the group intervention.

The increasing support for DBT as a treatment of depression in adults, the adolescent data on bipolar disorder, and basic research findings connecting bipolar disorder with high suicidality[7,30] and emotion dysregulation,[24,94] are indicators that DBT may be an effective treatment of adult bipolar disorder. Unfortunately, there is limited empirical research on DBT for adults with bipolar disorder. In one pilot study, when compared with a wait-list control group, a 12-week adaptation of DBT skills showed a trend toward significantly higher reductions in depression severity and improvement in emotional control in adults diagnosed with bipolar disorder.[95] Thus, more data are needed to support the use of DBT for bipolar disorder, especially in adults. Nevertheless, DBT is recognized as a promising option for the treatment of patients who are multi-diagnostic, difficult to treat, highly emotionally dysregulated, or engage in suicidal behavior.

COMMON PRINCIPLES FOR EFFECTIVE TREATMENT

Although the psychotherapy models available are based on very different theoretic foundations, effective treatments for bipolar depression converge on a few common principles. First, psychoeducation is a fundamental and primary step. In all empirically supported treatments presented, therapists educate patients about (1) the disorder, (2) cues and early warning signs of mood episodes, and (3) the importance of adherence to mood-stabilizing medication. Psychoeducation is such a crucial aspect that it can produce improvement on its own.[96] Second, patients with bipolar depression benefit from careful monitoring, increasing awareness, and understanding mood changes. Patients learn to keep track of their behavior and moods to identify *prodromal symptoms* (ie, early signs of a mood episode). In the presence of such cues, a stable daily routine helps patients intervene and prevent relapses. For example, disrupted sleep (eg, reduced need for sleep) is a prodromal cue that can indicate an increased risk for a mood episode; in this case, adhering to regular sleep cycles can prevent the onset of mania or depression.[97] Therefore, evidence-based psychotherapy protocols include maintaining regular routines in addition to psychoeducation. Finally, the importance of medication adherence is consistently emphasized. These common elements may serve as indicators to non–psychotherapy-trained providers about the quality of the psychotherapy intervention their patients might receive (**Box 6**).

Additional treatment recommendations come from research examining the importance of continuing the same type of psychotherapy versus having different treatments at different stages of bipolar disorder.[98] Empirical examinations found that maintaining the same treatment had a higher impact on preventing relapse than using different treatments during the acute and the remission phases of the disorder.[99] Therefore, it is recommended to follow a stable psychotherapy protocol with patients even through the different phases of the disorder.

The various psychotherapy protocols presented differ in the theoretic conceptualization regarding the cause and maintenance of depression. Nevertheless, currently it is unclear which of the hypothesized mechanisms provides the best approach to bipolar depression and whether moderators of treatment response (eg, sex, age) should be considered when offering different types of treatment.[10] In the absence of such research, the authors base our psychotherapy recommendations on primary complaints and how they match with existing approaches (see **Fig. 1**).

FUTURE MODELS

The psychotherapy models for bipolar depression presented earlier started as effective treatments for unipolar depression. Therefore, other empirically supported treatments for unipolar depression may offer promise for bipolar depression. Additional evidence-based protocols for unipolar depression that do not yet have research for bipolar depression are

1. Short-term psychodynamic psychotherapy[100–102]
2. Acceptance and commitment therapy[103–107]
3. Behavioral activation (BA)[108,109]
4. Cognitive behavioral analysis system of psychotherapy (CBASP)[110,111]
5. Functional analytical therapy[112–115]
6. Self-systems therapy[116]
7. The unified protocol (UP)[117–121]

The authors highlight the 3 approaches that they think show the most promise for bipolar depression.

Box 6
How to know if a therapist provides evidence-based psychotherapy for bipolar depression

1. Does the psychotherapy offered include psychoeducation about bipolar disorder?
2. Does the psychotherapy address medication compliance?
3. Is there a clear component of monitoring problems, mood, and/or medication?
4. Is establishing routines encouraged and directly addressed in therapy?
5. Can the therapist describe his or her training in the modality of the therapy offered?
6. Is the therapy offered an evidence-based treatment of bipolar depression or unipolar depression?

Behavioral Activation

BA[108,109] is based on the theory that depression develops because of insufficient positive reinforcement within the daily lives of those who become depressed.[122] Most appropriate for those patients whose primary complaint is anhedonia and amotivation, BA encourages patients to monitor their moods and actions in order to understand the relationship between what one does and how one feels. The main intervention is to develop strategies to increase pleasant (positively reinforcing), value-driven activities and decrease unpleasant activities in daily life. BA interventions have been shown to be effective in treating unipolar depression,[123] and the technique of scheduling and monitoring activities is strongly connected with reductions in depression severity.[124] BA's effectiveness with those with cognitive impairments[108,125] offers an advantage over CBT or MBCT; therefore, this intervention might meet the need of patients with bipolar depression who are too impaired to benefit from a highly cognitively based psychotherapy. See **Box 7** for a case example of using BA with a patient with bipolar depression.

Box 7
Case example

Robert was a 46-year-old man who was referred to the authors' clinic by the inpatient ward where he had been treated following a suicide attempt. When he presented for his initial evaluation, Robert was severely depressed, expressing hopelessness and suicidal ideation, although he was committed to safety and denied any intent to act on his ideation. Robert had previously been treated with psychodynamic psychotherapy by a psychiatrist in private practice. He described that he had been in and out of treatment, coming in at times of crisis and canceling or missing appointments during periods when he felt better. He reported that a recent loss of his employment had left him perceiving himself as an utter failure, a pervasive assessment he made regarding the totality of his life and his self. He described his marriage as rife with intense conflict, which he habitually responded to by submitting to his wife's demands or accusations and making apologies. He labeled himself a doormat and noted his humiliation when describing his patterns of coping.

Treatment began with a focus on value-driven behavioral activation, engaging him in activities, including gardening, hiking, and cooking, that brought him some joy—a marked contrast to the anhedonia he had been experiencing for many months. Robert began generating hope and built a sense of mastery by maintaining these activities regardless of mood. This first phase included monitoring of mood and activity and noting the fluctuations of mood that corresponded with interpersonal stressors and self-care, including eating regularly and maintaining a stable sleep schedule. The importance of medication compliance was emphasized, and self-efficacy was enhanced through strategies including phone reminders and visual reminders. Therapy also involved bringing his wife in and working with the couple on validation, conflict resolution, and understanding behavioral principles of reinforcement and shaping. DBT skills were incorporated to enhance his interpersonal effectiveness through building assertiveness and exploring boundary setting and maintenance; Robert practiced apologizing only if he was actually sorry and otherwise tolerating his wife's anger without making unnecessary apologies. Although these skills were challenging for him, he reported feeling empowered and competent, beginning to redefine his perception of his abilities and reducing his self-loathing. At this point, Robert became willing to reach out to friends whom he had been avoiding because of shame about his job loss and suicide attempt. These interactions provided positive reinforcement that supported his engagement in activities; the friends gave Robert feedback about his likable personal qualities, including kindness, humor, and creativity. This feedback increased his confidence and strengthened his ability to see that the self-loathing was rooted in his depression and the content of conflicts with his wife, allowing him to question the validity of such thoughts.

Cognitive Behavioral Analysis System of Psychotherapy

CBASP integrates behavioral and psychodynamic approaches into a treatment that is designed specifically for chronic depression.[111] The treatment encourages therapists to provide genuine feedback to patients as a way to shape in-session interpersonal behavior. The goal of this approach is to increase problem solving in important relationships through the use of situational analyses, which helps patient to closely examine their interpersonal behavior. In the largest RCT of CBASP, 681 chronically depressed patients were treated with nefazodone (an antidepressant), CBASP, or their combination.[110] CBASP alone had a 48% treatment response rate (as effective as nefazodone alone), whereas the combined treatment produced a significantly better response rate (72%). These results indicate that CBASP may be a promising treatment of individuals with bipolar disorder who tend to be in a chronically depressed or dysthymic (rather than euthymic) mood state when they are not in a hypomanic phase.

Unified Protocol

Based on observations that there is a great deal of overlap between the different anxiety and mood disorders, Barlow and colleagues[118] have been developing a transdiagnostic treatment approach that includes 8 treatment modules focusing on psychoeducation, emotional awareness and tolerance, cognitive and behavioral strategies, and relapse prevention.[121] This approach has been shown to be efficacious for treating anxiety with comorbid depression (but excluding bipolar) in a recent RCT.[120] Although empirical research with patients with bipolar disorder is needed, the UP may be a useful option when patients with bipolar disorder are also diagnosed with several anxiety disorders.

SUMMARY

These additional approaches offer promise for treatment of bipolar depression. The authors encourage researchers to evaluate their application and efficacy with bipolar depression. In addition, mental health care providers who have found other evidence-based treatments unsuccessful are also encouraged to use some of these additional protocols in their treatment plans.

REFERENCES

1. Judd LL, Akiskal HS. The prevalence and disability of bipolar spectrum disorders in the US population: re-analysis of the ECA database taking into account subthreshold cases. J Affect Disord 2003;73(1–2):123–31.
2. Geddes JR, Burgess S, Hawton K, et al. Long-term lithium therapy for bipolar disorder: systematic review and meta-analysis of randomized controlled trials. Am J Psychiatry 2004;161(2):217–22.
3. Geddes JR, Miklowitz DJ. Treatment of bipolar disorder. Lancet 2013;381: 1672–82.
4. Judd LL, Akiskal HS, Schettler PJ, et al. The long-term natural history of the weekly symptomatic status of bipolar I disorder. Arch Gen Psychiatry 2002; 59(6):530–7.
5. Judd LL, Schettler PJ, Akiskal HS, et al. Long-term symptomatic status of bipolar I vs. bipolar II disorders. Int J Neuropsychopharmacol 2003;6(2):127–37.
6. Hoertel N, Limosin F, Leleu H. Poor longitudinal continuity of care is associated with an increased mortality rate among patients with mental disorders: results from the French National Health Insurance Reimbursement Database. Eur Psychiatry 2014;29:358–64.

7. Hoertel N, Franco S, Wall MM, et al. Mental disorders and risk of suicide attempt: a national prospective study. Mol Psychiatry 2015;20:718–26.

8. Kessler RC, Akiskal HS, Angst J, et al. Validity of the assessment of bipolar spectrum disorders in the WHO CIDI 3.0. J Affect Disord 2006;96(3):259–69.

9. Altshuler LL, Gitlin MJ, Mintz J, et al. Subsyndromal depression is associated with functional impairment in patients with bipolar disorder. J Clin Psychiatry 2002;63(9):807–11.

10. Hoertel N, de Maricourt P, Gorwood P. Novel routes to bipolar disorder drug discovery. Expert Opin Drug Discov 2013;8:907–18.

11. Sachs GS. Treatment-resistant bipolar depression. Psychiatr Clin North Am 1996;19(2):215–36.

12. Gitlin M. Treatment-resistant bipolar disorder. Mol Psychiatry 2006;11(3): 227–40.

13. Gershon S, Soares JC. Current therapeutic profile of lithium. Arch Gen Psychiatry 1997;54(1):16–20.

14. Hoertel N, Le Strat Y, Lavaud P, et al. Generalizability of clinical trial results for bipolar disorder to community samples: findings from the National Epidemiologic Survey on Alcohol and Related Conditions. J Clin Psychiatry 2013;74: 265–70.

15. Zaretsky AE, Rizvi S, Parikh SV. How well do psychosocial interventions work in bipolar disorder? Can J Psychiatry 2007;52(1):14.

16. Hoertel N, Le Strat Y, Limosin F, et al. Prevalence of subthreshold hypomania and impact on internal validity of RCTs for major depressive disorder: results from a national epidemiological sample. PLoS One 2013;8:e55448.

17. Hoertel N, Le Strat Y, Angst J, et al. Subthreshold bipolar disorder in a U.S. national representative sample: prevalence, correlates and perspectives for psychiatric nosography. J Affect Disord 2013;146(3):338–47.

18. Miklowitz DJ. A review of evidence-based psychosocial interventions for bipolar disorder. J Clin Psychiat 2006;67:28–33.

19. Hollon SD, Munoz RF, Barlow DH, et al. Psychosocial intervention development for the prevention and treatment of depression: promoting innovation and increasing access. Biol Psychiatry 2002;52(6):610–30.

20. DeRubeis RJ, Siegle GJ, Hollon SD. Cognitive therapy versus medication for depression: treatment outcomes and neural mechanisms. Nat Rev Neurosci 2008;9(10):788–96.

21. First MB, Spitzer RL, Gibbon M, et al. Structured clinical interview for DSM-IV axis I disorders—patient edition (SCID-I/P, version 2.0). New York: Biometrics Research Department; State Psychiatric Institute; 1995.

22. Hirschfeld RM, Williams JB, Spitzer RL, et al. Development and validation of a screening instrument for bipolar spectrum disorder: the Mood Disorder Questionnaire. Am J Psychiatry 2000;157(11):1873–5.

23. Perlis RH, Brown E, Baker RW, et al. Clinical features of bipolar depression versus major depressive disorder in large multicenter trials. Am J Psychiatry 2006;163(2):225–31.

24. Perugi G, Akiskal HS, Lattanzi L, et al. The high prevalence of "soft" bipolar (II) features in atypical depression. Compr Psychiatry 1998;39(2):63–71.

25. Hantouche EG, Akiskal HS. Bipolar II vs. unipolar depression: psychopathologic differentiation by dimensional measures. J Affect Disord 2005;84(2–3): 127–32.

26. Mitchell PB, Goodwin GM, Johnson GF, et al. Diagnostic guidelines for bipolar depression: a probabilistic approach. Bipolar Disord 2008;10(1 Pt 2):144–52.

27. Mitchell PB, Wilhelm K, Parker G, et al. The clinical features of bipolar depression: a comparison with matched major depressive disorder patients. J Clin Psychiatry 2001;62(3):212–6.

28. Mitchell PB, Malhi GS. Bipolar depression: phenomenological overview and clinical characteristics. Bipolar Disord 2004;6(6):530–9.

29. Parker G, Roy K, Wilhelm K, et al. The nature of bipolar depression: implications for the definition of melancholia. J Affect Disord 2000;59(3):217–24.

30. Moreno C, Hasin DS, Arango C, et al. Depression in bipolar disorder versus major depressive disorder: results from the National Epidemiologic Survey on Alcohol and Related Conditions. Bipolar Disord 2012;14(3):271–82.

31. Angst J, Cui L, Swendsen J, et al. Major depressive disorder with subthreshold bipolarity in the National Comorbidity Survey Replication. Am J Psychiatry 2010; 167:1194–201.

32. Zutshi A, Kamath P, Reddy YCJ. Bipolar and nonbipolar obsessive-compulsive disorder: a clinical exploration. Compr Psychiatry 2007;48:245–51.

33. Toniolo RA, Caetano SC, da Silva PV, et al. Clinical significance of lifetime panic disorder in the course of bipolar disorder type I. Compr Psychiatry 2009;50:9–12.

34. Nierenberg AA, Ostacher MJ, Calabrese JR, et al. Treatment-resistant bipolar depression: a STEP-BD equipoise randomized effectiveness trial of antidepressant augmentation with lamotrigine, inositol, or risperidone. Am J Psychiatry 2006;163:210–6.

35. Beck JS. Cognitive behavior therapy: basics and beyond. Guilford Press; 2011.

36. Beck A. Cognitive therapy of depression. New York: Guilford Press; 1979.

37. Basco MR, Rush AJ. Cognitive-behavioral therapy for bipolar disorder. New York: Guilford Press; 2005.

38. Lam DH, Jones SH, Hayward P. Cognitive therapy for bipolar disorder: a therapist's guide to concepts, methods and practice. West Sussex, UK: Wiley-Blackwell; 2010.

39. Scott J. Cognitive therapy as an adjunct to medication in bipolar disorder. Br J Psychiatry Suppl 2001;178:s164–8.

40. Gregory VL. Cognitive-behavioral therapy for depression in bipolar disorder: a meta-analysis. J Evid Based Soc Work 2010;7:269–79.

41. Ball JR, Mitchell PB, Corry JC, et al. A randomized controlled trial of cognitive therapy for bipolar disorder: focus on long-term change. J Clin Psychiatry 2006;67:277–86.

42. Zaretsky AE, Segal ZV, Gemar M. Cognitive therapy for bipolar depression: a pilot study. Can J Psychiatry 1999;44:491–4.

43. Scott J, Paykel E, Morriss R, et al. Cognitive-behavioural therapy for severe and recurrent bipolar disorders: randomised controlled trial. Br J Psychiatry 2006; 188:313–20.

44. Miklowitz DJ, Otto MW, Frank E, et al. Psychosocial treatments for bipolar depression: a 1-year randomized trial from the systematic treatment enhancement program. Arch Gen Psychiatry 2007;64(4):419–26.

45. Miklowitz DJ, Ph D, Otto MW, et al. Intensive psychosocial intervention enhances functioning in patients with bipolar depression: results from a 9-month randomized controlled trial. Am J Psychiatry 2007;164(9):1340–7.

46. Patelis-Siotis I, Young LT, Robb JC, et al. Group cognitive behavioral therapy for bipolar disorder: a feasibility and effectiveness study. J Affect Disord 2001;65: 145–53.

47. Costa RT, Cheniaux E, Rangé BP, et al. Group cognitive behavior therapy for bipolar disorder can improve the quality of life. Braz J Med Biol Res 2012;45:862–8.

48. Costa RTD, Cheniaux E, Rosaes PAL, et al. The effectiveness of cognitive behavioral group therapy in treating bipolar disorder: a randomized controlled study. Rev Bras Psiquiatr (São Paulo, Brazil: 1999) 2011;33:144–9.

49. Lam DH, Watkins ER, Hayward P, et al. A randomized controlled study of cognitive therapy for relapse prevention for bipolar affective disorder. Arch Gen Psychiatry 2003;60:145–52.

50. Lam DH, Hayward P, Watkins ER, et al. Relapse prevention in patients with bipolar disorder: cognitive therapy outcome after 2 years. Am J Psychiatry 2005;162:324–9.

51. Butzlaff RL, Hooley JM. Expressed emotion and psychiatric relapse: a meta-analysis. Arch Gen Psychiatry 1998;55:547–52.

52. Miklowitz DJ, Goldstein MJ, Nuechterlein KH. Verbal interactions in the families of schizophrenic and bipolar affective patients. J Abnorm Psychol 1995;104:268–76.

53. Miklowitz DJ, Goldstein MJ. Behavioral family treatment for patients with bipolar affective disorder. Behav Modif 1990;14:457–89.

54. Miklowitz DJ. Adjunctive psychotherapy for bipolar disorder: state of the evidence. Am J Psychiatry 2008;165:1408–19.

55. Miklowitz DJ, George EL, Richards JA, et al. A randomized study of family-focused psychoeducation and pharmacotherapy in the outpatient management of bipolar disorder. Arch Gen Psychiatry 2003;60:904–12.

56. Simoneau TL, Miklowitz DJ, Richards JA, et al. Bipolar disorder and family communication: effects of a psychoeducational treatment program. J Abnorm Psychol 1999;108(4):588–97.

57. Miklowitz DJ, Axelson DA, Birmaher B, et al. Family-focused treatment for adolescents with bipolar disorder: results of a 2-year randomized trial. Arch Gen Psychiatry 2008;65(9):1053–61.

58. Rea MM, Tompson MC, Miklowitz DJ, et al. Family-focused treatment versus individual treatment for bipolar disorder: results of a randomized clinical trial. J Consult Clin Psychol 2003;71:482–92.

59. Frank E, Swartz HA, Kupfer DJ. Interpersonal and social rhythm therapy: managing the chaos of bipolar disorder. Biol Psychiatry 2000;48:593–604.

60. Leibenluft E, Albert PS, Rosenthal NE, et al. Relationship between sleep and mood in patients with rapid-cycling bipolar disorder. Psychiatry Res 1996;63(2–3):161–8.

61. Klerman GL, Weissman MM, Rounsaville BJ, et al. Interpersonal psychotherapy of depression. New York: Basic Books Inc; 1984.

62. de Mello MF, de Jesus Mari J, Bacaltchuk J, et al. A systematic review of research findings on the efficacy of interpersonal therapy for depressive disorders. Eur Arch Psychiatry Clin Neurosci 2005;255:75–82.

63. Frank E, Kupfer DJ, Thase ME, et al. Two-year outcomes for interpersonal and social rhythm therapy in individuals with bipolar I disorder. Arch Gen Psychiatry 2005;62:996–1004.

64. Frank E, Soreca I, Swartz HA, et al. The role of interpersonal and social rhythm therapy in improving occupational functioning in patients with bipolar I disorder. Am J Psychiatry 2008;165(12):1559–65.

65. Swartz HA, Frank E, Frankel DR, et al. Psychotherapy as monotherapy for the treatment of bipolar II depression: a proof of concept study. Bipolar Disord 2009;11(1):89–94.

66. Bouwkamp CG, de Kruiff ME, van Troost TM, et al. Interpersonal and social rhythm group therapy for patients with bipolar disorder. Int J Group Psychother 2013;63(1):97–115.

67. Hoberg AA, Ponto J, Nelson PJ, et al. Group interpersonal and social rhythm therapy for bipolar depression. Perspect Psychiatr Care 2013;49(4):226–34.
68. Segal ZV, Williams JMG, Teasdale JD. Mindfulness-based cognitive therapy for depression. New York: Guilford Press; 2012.
69. Deckersbach T, Hölzel B, Eisner L, et al. Mindfulness-based cognitive therapy for bipolar disorder. New York: Guilford Press; 2014.
70. Chiesa A, Serretti A. Mindfulness based cognitive therapy for psychiatric disorders: a systematic review and meta-analysis. Psychiatry Res 2011;187: 441–53.
71. Fjorback LO, Arendt M, Ornbol E, et al. Mindfulness-based stress reduction and mindfulness-based cognitive therapy - a systematic review of randomized controlled trials. Acta Psychiatr Scand 2011;124:102–19.
72. Piet J, Hougaard E. The effect of mindfulness-based cognitive therapy for prevention of relapse in recurrent major depressive disorder: a systematic review and meta-analysis. Clin Psychol Rev 2011;31:1032–40.
73. Williams JM, Alatiq Y, Crane C, et al. Mindfulness-based cognitive therapy (MBCT) in bipolar disorder: preliminary evaluation of immediate effects on between-episode functioning. J Affect Disord 2008;107(1–3):275–9.
74. Deckersbach T, Holzel BK, Eisner LR, et al. Mindfulness-based cognitive therapy for nonremitted patients with bipolar disorder. CNS Neurosci Ther 2012; 18(2):133–41.
75. Miklowitz DJ, Alatiq Y, Goodwin GM, et al. A pilot study of mindfulness-based cognitive therapy for bipolar disorder. Int J Cog Ther 2009;2(4):373–82.
76. Stange JP, Eisner LR, Hölzel BK, et al. Mindfulness-based cognitive therapy for bipolar disorder: effects on cognitive functioning. J Psychiatr Pract 2011;17: 410–9.
77. Perich T, Manicavasagar V, Mitchell PB, et al. A randomized controlled trial of mindfulness-based cognitive therapy for bipolar disorder. Acta Psychiatr Scand 2013;127(5):333–43.
78. Howells FM, Laurie Rauch HG, Ives-Deliperi VL, et al. Mindfulness based cognitive therapy may improve emotional processing in bipolar disorder: pilot ERP and HRV study. Metab Brain Dis 2014;29(2):367–75.
79. Howells FM, Ives-Deliperi VL, Horn NR, et al. Mindfulness based cognitive therapy improves frontal control in bipolar disorder: a pilot EEG study. BMC Psychiatry 2012;12(1):15–23.
80. Ives-Deliperi VL, Howells F, Stein DJ, et al. The effects of mindfulness-based cognitive therapy in patients with bipolar disorder: a controlled functional MRI investigation. J Affect Disord 2013;150(3):1152–7.
81. Linehan M. Cognitive-behavioral treatment of borderline personality disorder. New York: Guilford Press; 1993.
82. Linehan MM. Skills training manual for treating borderline personality disorder, vol. xii. New York: Guilford Press; 1993.
83. Crowell SE, Beauchaine TP, Linehan MM. A biosocial developmental model of borderline personality: elaborating and extending Linehan's theory. Psychol Bull 2009;135(3):495–510.
84. Linehan MM, Comtois KA, Brown MZ, et al. Suicide Attempt Self-Injury Interview (SASII): development, reliability, and validity of a scale to assess suicide attempts and intentional self-injury. Psychol Assess 2006;18(3):303–12.
85. Neacsiu AD, Bohus M, Linehan MM. Dialectical behavior therapy: an intervention for emotion dysregulation. In: Gross JJ, editor. Handbook of emotion regulation. 2 edition. New York: The Guilford Press; 2013. p. 491–508.

86. Kring AM, Werner KH. Emotion regulation and psychopathology. In: Philippot P, Feldman RS, editors. The regulation of emotion. Mahwah (NJ): Lawrence Erlbaum Associates Publishers; 2004. p. 359–85.

87. Neacsiu AD, Eberle JW, Kramer R, et al. Dialectical behavior therapy skills for transdiagnostic emotion dysregulation: a pilot randomized controlled trial. Behav Res Ther 2014;59:40–51.

88. Lynch TR, Morse JQ, Mendelson T, et al. Dialectical behavior therapy for depressed older adults: a randomized pilot study. Am J Geriatr Psychiatry 2003;11(1):33–45.

89. Harley R, Sprich S, Safren S, et al. Adaptation of dialectical behavior therapy skills training group for treatment-resistant depression. J Nerv Ment Dis 2008; 196(2):136–43.

90. Ritschel LA, Cheavens JS, Nelson J. Dialectical behavior therapy in an intensive outpatient program with a mixed-diagnostic sample. J Clin Psychol 2012;68(3): 221–35.

91. Goldstein TR, Axelson DA, Birmaher B, et al. Dialectical behavior therapy for adolescents with bipolar disorder: a 1-year open trial. J Am Acad Child Psychiatry 2007;46(7):820–30.

92. Goldstein TR, Fersch-Podrat RK, Rivera M, et al. Dialectical behavior therapy for adolescents with bipolar disorder: results from a pilot randomized trial. J Child Adolesc Psychopharmacol 2015;25(2):140–9.

93. Miller AL, Rathus JH, Linehan MM. Dialectical behavior therapy with suicidal adolescents. New York: Guilford Press; 2006.

94. Gruber J, Kogan A, Mennin D, et al. Real-world emotion? An experience-sampling approach to emotion experience and regulation in bipolar I disorder. J Abnorm Psy 2013;122(4):971–83.

95. Van Dijk S, Jeffrey J, Katz MR. A randomized, controlled, pilot study of dialectical behavior therapy skills in a psychoeducational group for individuals with bipolar disorder. J Affect Disord 2013;145(3):386–93.

96. Perry A, Tarrier N, Morriss R, et al. Randomised controlled trial of efficacy of teaching patients with bipolar disorder to identify early symptoms of relapse and obtain treatment. BMJ (Clinical Research ed) 1999;318:149–53.

97. Harvey AG. Sleep and circadian rhythms in bipolar disorder: seeking synchrony, harmony, and regulation. Am J Psychiatry 2008;165:820–9.

98. Swartz HA, Frank E. Psychotherapy for bipolar depression: a phase-specific treatment strategy? Bipolar Disord 2001;3(1):11–22.

99. Frank E, Swartz HA, Mallinger AG, et al. Adjunctive psychotherapy for bipolar disorder: effects of changing treatment modality. J Abnorm Psychol 1999;108: 579–87.

100. Leichsenring F. Comparative effects of short-term psychodynamic psychotherapy and cognitive-behavioral therapy in depression: a meta-analytic approach. Clin Psychol Rev 2001;21(3):401–19.

101. Leichsenring F, Rabung S. Effectiveness of long-term psychodynamic psychotherapy: a meta-analysis. JAMA 2008;300(13):1551–65.

102. Leichsenring F, Rabung S, Leibing E. The efficacy of short-term psychodynamic psychotherapy in specific psychiatric disorders: a meta-analysis. Arch Gen Psychiatry 2004;61:1208–16.

103. Hayes SC, Luoma JB, Bond FW, et al. Acceptance and commitment therapy: model, processes and outcomes. Behav Res Ther 2006;44(1):1–25.

104. Markanday S, Data-Franco J, Dyson L, et al. Acceptance and commitment therapy for treatment-resistant depression. Aust N Z J Psychiatry 2012;46(12):1198–9.

105. Mohabbat-Bahar S, Maleki-Rizi F, Akbari ME, et al. Effectiveness of group training based on acceptance and commitment therapy on anxiety and depression of women with breast cancer. Iran J Cancer Prev 2015;8(2):71–6.

106. Karlin BE, Walser RD, Yesavage J, et al. Effectiveness of acceptance and commitment therapy for depression: comparison among older and younger veterans. Aging Ment Health 2013;17(5):555–63.

107. Heffner JL, McClure JB, Mull KE, et al. Acceptance and commitment therapy and nicotine patch for smokers with bipolar disorder: preliminary evaluation of in-person and telephone-delivered treatment. Bipolar Disord 2015;17(5): 560–6.

108. Dimidjian S, Hollon SD, Dobson KS, et al. Randomized trial of behavioral activation, cognitive therapy, and antidepressant medication in the acute treatment of adults with major depression. J Consult Clin Psychol 2006;74(4):658–70.

109. Jacobson NS, Martell CR, Dimidjian S. Behavioral activation treatment for depression: returning to contextual roots. Clin Psychol Sci Pract 2001;8(3): 255–70.

110. Keller MB, McCullough JP, Klein DN, et al. A comparison of nefazodone, the cognitive behavioral-analysis system of psychotherapy, and their combination for the treatment of chronic depression. N Engl J Med 2000;342(20):1462–70.

111. McCullough JP Jr. Treatment for chronic depression: cognitive behavioral analysis system of psychotherapy (CBASP). New York: Guilford Press; 2003.

112. Kohlenberg RJ, Kanter JW, Bolling MY, et al. Enhancing cognitive therapy for depression with functional analytic psychotherapy: treatment guidelines and empirical findings. Cog Beh Pract 2002;9(3):213–29.

113. Kohlenberg RJ, Tsai M. Functional analytic psychotherapy: a guide for creating intense and curative therapeutic relationships. New York: Plenum Press; 1991.

114. Kohlenberg RJ, Tsai M. Improving cognitive therapy for depression with functional analytic psychotherapy: theory and case study. Behav Anal 1994;17(2): 305–19.

115. Kanter JW, Landes SJ, Busch AM, et al. The effect of contingent reinforcement on target variables in outpatient psychotherapy for depression: a successful and unsuccessful case using functional analytic psychotherapy. J Appl Behav Anal 2006;39(4):463–7.

116. Strauman TJ, Vieth AZ, Merrill KA, et al. Self-system therapy as an intervention for self-regulatory dysfunction in depression: a randomized comparison with cognitive therapy. J Consult Clin Psychol 2006;74(2):367–76.

117. Barlow DH, Allen LB, Choate ML. Toward a unified treatment for emotional disorders. Behav Ther 2004;35(2):205–30.

118. Barlow DH, Farchione TJ, Fairholme CP, et al. Unified protocol for transdiagnostic treatment of emotional disorders: therapist guide. New York: Oxford University Press; 2011.

119. Ehrenreich JT, Goldstein CM, Wright LR, et al. Development of a unified protocol for the treatment of emotional disorders in youth. Child Fam Behav Ther 2009; 31(1):20–37.

120. Farchione TJ, Fairholme CP, Ellard KK, et al. Unified protocol for transdiagnostic treatment of emotional disorders: a randomized controlled trial. Behav Ther 2012;43(3):666–78.

121. Wilamowska ZA, Thompson-Hollands J, Fairholme CP, et al. Conceptual background, development, and preliminary data from the unified protocol for transdiagnostic treatment of emotional disorders. Depress Anxiety 2010;27(10): 882–90.

122. Lewinsohn PM. A behavioral approach to depression. In: Friedman RJ, Katz MM, editors. The psychology of depression: contemporary theory and research. Washington, DC: Wiley; 1974. p. 157–85.
123. Mazzucchelli T, Kane R, Rees C. Behavioral activation treatments for depression in adults: a meta-analysis and review. Clin Psychol Sci Pract 2009;16: 383–411.
124. Cuijpers P, van Straten A, Warmerdam L. Behavioral activation treatments of depression: a meta-analysis. Clin Psychol Rev 2007;27:318–26.
125. Teri L, Logsdon RG, Uomoto J, et al. Behavioral treatment of depression in dementia patients: a controlled clinical trial. J Gerontol B Psychol Sci Soc Sci 1997; 52(4):P159–66.
126. First MB, Williams JB, Karg RL. Structured clinical interview for DSM-5 disorders (research version: SCID-5-RV). Washington, DC: American Psychiatric Publishing; 2015.
127. Endicott J, Spitzer RL. A diagnostic interview: the schedule for affective disorders and schizophrenia. Arch Gen Psychiatry 1978;35(7):837–44.
128. Hamilton M. A rating scale for depression. J Neurol Neurosurg Psychiatry 1960; 23(1):56–62.
129. Beck AT, Ward C, Mendelson M. Beck depression inventory (BDI). Arch Gen Psychiatry 1961;4(6):561–71.
130. Beck A, Steer R, Brown G. Manual for the BDI-II. San Antonio (TX): Psychological Corporation; 1996.
131. Löwe B, Kroenke K, Herzog W, et al. Measuring depression outcome with a brief self-report instrument: sensitivity to change of the patient health questionnaire (PHQ-9). J Affect Disord 2004;81(1):61–6.
132. Spitzer RL, Kroenke K, Williams JB. Validation and utility of a self-report version of PRIME-MD: the PHQ primary care study. Primary care evaluation of mental disorders. Patient health questionnaire. JAMA 1999;282(18):1737–44.
133. Bech P, Rafaelsen O, Kramp P, et al. The mania rating scale: scale construction and inter-observer agreement. Neuropharmacology 1978;17(6):430–1.
134. Hollon SD, Kendall PC. Cognitive self-statements in depression: development of an automatic thoughts questionnaire. Cogn Ther Res 1980;4(4):383–95.
135. Wcissman A, Beck AT. Development and validation of the Dysfunctional Attitude Scale. Paper presented at the annual convention of the Association for Advancement of Behavior Therapy. Chicago, 1978.
136. Beck AT, Weissman A, Lester D, et al. The measurement of pessimism: the hopelessness scale. J Consult Clin Psychol 1974;42(6):861.
137. Nolen-Hoeksema S, Morrow J. A prospective study of depression and posttraumatic stress symptoms after a natural disaster: the 1989 Loma Prieta Earthquake. J Pers Soc Psychol 1991;61(1):115–21.
138. Vaughn C, Leff J. The measurement of expressed emotion in the families of psychiatric patients. Br J Soc Clin Psychol 1976;15(2):157–65.
139. Hahlweg K, Reisner L, Kohli G, et al. Development and validity of a new system to analyze interpersonal communication (KPI: Kategoriensystem für partnerschaftliche Interaktion). In: Hahlweg K, Jacobson NS, editors. Marital Interaction: Analysis and Modification. New York: Guilford Press; 1984. p. 182–98.
140. Magaña AB, Goldstein MJ, Karno M, et al. A brief method for assessing expressed emotion in relatives of psychiatric patients. Psychiatry Res 1986; 17(3):203–12.
141. Monk TK, Flaherty JF, Frank E, et al. The social rhythm metric: an instrument to quantify the daily rhythms of life. J Nerv Ment Dis 1990;178(2):120–6.

142. Weissman MM, Bothwell S. Assessment of social adjustment by patient self-report. Arch Gen Psychiatry 1976;33(9):1111–5.
143. Horowitz LM, Rosenberg SE, Baer BA, et al. Inventory of interpersonal problems: psychometric properties and clinical applications. J Consult Clin Psychol 1988;56(6):885–92.
144. Brown TA, Barlow DH, Di Nardo PA. Anxiety disorders interview schedule adult version: client interview schedule. New York: Oxford University Press; 1994.
145. Beck AT, Steer RA. Manual for the Beck anxiety inventory. San Antonio (TX): Psychological Corporation; 1990.
146. Gratz KL, Roemer L. Multidimensional assessment of emotion regulation and dysregulation: development, factor structure, and initial validation of the difficulties in emotion regulation scale. J Psychopathol Behav Assess 2004;26(1): 41–54.
147. Bond FW, Hayes SC, Baer RA, et al. Preliminary psychometric properties of the acceptance and action questionnaire–II: a revised measure of psychological inflexibility and experiential avoidance. Behav Ther 2011;42(4):676–88.
148. Hayes S, Strosahl K, Wilson K, et al. Acceptance and action questionnaire. Psychol Rec 1996;5(4):553–78.
149. Garnefski N, Kraaij V. Cognitive emotion regulation questionnaire–development of a short 18-item version (CERQ-short). Pers Individ Dif 2006;41(6):1045–53.
150. Baer RA, Smith GT, Allen KB. Assessment of mindfulness by self-report the Kentucky inventory of mindfulness skills. Assessment 2004;11(3):191–206.
151. Brown KW, Ryan RM. The benefits of being present: mindfulness and its role in psychological well-being. J Pers Soc Psychol 2003;84(4):822.

Bipolar Depression
Pregnancy, Postpartum, and Lactation

Marla F. Wald, MD[a],*, Andrew J. Muzyk, PharmD[b], Drue Clark, PharmD, BCACP[c]

KEYWORDS

• Bipolar depression • Pregnancy • Postpartum • Lactation

KEY POINTS

• Medication management of bipolar depression in pregnancy and lactation is best done by assessing each patient's and family's needs in detail.

• Keeping pregnant patients as psychiatrically stable as possible is the most important principle for clinicians, in conjunction with assessing the various risks and benefits of the medications.

• There is no 100% risk-free situation for patients with psychiatric illness because both illness and medications present potential risks to mother and baby.

• Clinicians serve these patients best by being as transparent as possible about the risk/benefit analysis of each patient's situation with the realization that ultimately the decisions are made by the patient and family.

INTRODUCTION

Pharmacologic treatment of bipolar depression becomes additionally complex during the continuum of pregnancy and the postpartum period for multiple reasons. First, misdiagnosis of bipolar depressive episodes as unipolar depression is common. Mistakenly treating symptoms as if they were part of only a unipolar depression risks triggering manic and psychotic symptoms with documented severe outcomes, potentially including baby harm thoughts, suicide, and (more rarely) infanticide. The diagnosis is often made more difficult due to the inherent disruptions to sleep, energy, and appetite, both before and after delivery. Therefore, treatment begins with an accurate diagnosis, differentiating not only between unipolar and bipolar depressions but also between the subtypes of bipolar disorder (bipolar I disorder, bipolar II disorder, and mixed bipolar disorder). Second, common medications used in bipolar illness

---

[a] Department of Psychiatry and Behavioral Sciences, Duke University Medical Center, Civitan Building, 2213 Elba Street, Durham, NC 27705, USA; [b] Campbell University College of Pharmacy and Health Sciences, Buies Creek, NC, USA; [c] Mission Health Outpatient Clinical Pharmacy Services, Asheville, NC, USA
* Corresponding author.
E-mail address: marla.wald@duke.edu

Psychiatr Clin N Am 39 (2016) 57–74
http://dx.doi.org/10.1016/j.psc.2015.10.002
0193-953X/16/$ – see front matter © 2016 Elsevier Inc. All rights reserved.

may cause adverse effects to the developing fetus. Thus, decisions for treatment in the present episode may reverberate for a lifetime, both parents' and child's.

The risks of fetal and maternal exposure to untreated illness must be weighed against the risks of exposure to medications in terms of teratogenicity, obstetric complications, birth outcomes, neonatal outcomes, and neurodevelopmental outcomes. Because of this complexity, clinicians often decide that pharmacologic treatment is incompatible in a pregnant bipolar depressed patient and may recommend discontinuation of bipolar medications. Untreated bipolar depression, however, may also lead to unfortunate outcomes. Furthermore, the impact of the illness and its treatment is not limited to the patients themselves but also includes the fetus or newborn and a patient's other children, spouse, and extended family. These considerations lead to complicated decision-making algorithms for a treating clinician.

Whereas treatment of pregnant women with bipolar disorder has been a neglected area of study in the past, there has been increased attention over the past decade to studies identifying and treating perinatal bipolar disorder.[1–5] With knowledgeable attention to the clinical picture and available evidence, bipolar depression can be managed with a positive outcome.

This article addresses pharmacologic approaches to the treatment of bipolar depression during pregnancy and the postpartum period. The pros and cons of currently available pharmacologic treatments are reviewed and clinical recommendations for the management of medications throughout pregnancy, postpartum, and lactation are provided.

EPIDEMIOLOGY
Bipolar Rates in Women

The National Comorbidity Survey has estimated the lifetime prevalence rate of bipolar disorder at 3.9%[6] among the adult population. In general, the prevalence rate of bipolar I disorder is similar between men and women. According to the World Health Organization,[7] however, the burden of depression is 50% higher in women than in men and is one of the leading causes of disease burden in women across the globe. Women with bipolar disorder tend to experience more depressive episodes during the active phases of illness compared with men.[4,8,9] Furthermore, although the prevalence rate of bipolar I disorder is similar in men and women, the rate of bipolar II disorder is higher in women, and depressive symptoms are 30 times more prevalent than hypomanic symptoms.[4,10–12]

Bipolar Rates During Pregnancy and the Postpartum Period

Pregnancy and the postpartum period is the most vulnerable time in a woman's life for mental health problems or psychiatric hospitalization. This is especially true for women with bipolar disorder. Prospective studies documenting bipolar episodes in pregnancy have reported that up to 70% of women may have an acute mood episode during pregnancy,[13,14] although the postpartum phase may be the most vulnerable.[1] Viguera and colleagues[5] evaluated pregnancy outcomes in 1162 women (2252 pregnancies) with mood disorders (bipolar I disorder – 479 pregnancies, bipolar II disorder – 641 pregnancies, and major depressive disorder [MDD] recurrent – 1132 pregnancies). Of the bipolar women, 23% of them had a mood episode during pregnancy, whereas 52% had an episode during the postpartum period. Depression was the most frequent morbidity. The risk for depression was consistently higher in bipolar patients compared with unipolar depression.[5] Furthermore, there is also evidence that women who have had previous diagnoses of premenstrual syndrome and premenstrual dysphoric disorder, which identify them as sensitive to hormonal changes, are at higher risk for MDD or bipolar disorder episodes during pregnancy and postpartum.[15]

In a prospective cohort study of 1212 women with bipolar disorder in the United Kingdom, 25% of women with bipolar I had a depressive episode either in pregnancy or postpartum.[16] Similar to previous studies, the onset of mood episodes was less common in pregnancy than during the postpartum period. Women with bipolar II disorder had fewer depressive episodes than bipolar I women, but the rate still remained high. Women with bipolar II, however, were more likely to have depressive episodes during pregnancy and in the late postpartum time compared with women with bipolar I, who were more likely to have episodes of depression in the immediate first 4 weeks postpartum.[16]

Rates of Relapse with Sudden Stopping of Medications

Viguera and colleagues[17] found that after discontinuing lithium, pregnant and nonpregnant women had similar recurrence rates within 40 weeks (52%); however, during weeks 41 to 50 after discontinuation, women in the postpartum period were 2.9 times more likely to have episodes compared with the other women. Furthermore, rapid discontinuation was associated with greater likelihood of recurrences than gradual discontinuation.

In a prospective study of 86 pregnant women with bipolar disorder, Viguera and colleagues[14] found relapse rates of 71% during pregnancy, most of which were depressive episodes. If the mood stabilizer was discontinued, the woman was twice as likely to have an episode, it started 4 times more quickly, and it lasted 5 times as long. Abrupt discontinuation amplified these findings. Recurrence occurred 11 times more quickly than for those who slowly tapered their mood stabilizer.

Risks to Fetus and Neonate with Untreated Maternal Diagnoses of Bipolar Disorder

It is difficult to assess the impact of bipolar disorder, much less untreated bipolar disorder, on fetuses during pregnancy. Most of the data come from registration databases. These are population-based cohorts, as opposed to randomized clinical trials, in which there is little control over other maternal variables, such as smoking, drug use, adverse lifestyles, comorbid conditions, genetic/family history of birth defects, and birth outcomes. Current evidence related to untreated bipolar disorder, however, indicates numerous unfavorable outcomes to mothers and babies These may include placental abruption/abnormalities, preeclampsia, preterm delivery, intrauterine growth restriction, low birth weight, fetal distress, low Apgar scores, congenital defects, stillbirths, and neurodevelopmental difficulties.[18–20] Most of the data used to guide perinatal clinical decision making have been gathered from registries, retrospective chart reviews, and naturalistic cohort and case studies. Safety data about various medications in the perinatal time frame come primarily from the absence of negative reports rather than from the presence of positive studies.

MEDICATIONS
Explanation of the Food and Drug Administration Rating System for Medication Effects in Pregnancy

The current Food and Drug Administration (FDA) teratogenic risk classification system was established in 1979 and, although it has been under proposed revision since 2008, the structure of the current system remains unchanged. The system originated in response to the 1960s thalidomide controversy and rated medications according to static categories of risk A, B, C, D, and X (**Table 1**). In 2004, a lactation risk category

Table 1
Medication impact during pregnancy

Category	Medication	Teratogenic Risk/ Lactation Risk	Comments
Mood stabilizers	Lithium	D/L4	In TM1, slight increased risk of Ebstein anomaly but low absolute risk overall. D/C at start of contractions to avoid toxicity and transient floppy infant. Avoid during lactation if possible due to high excretion in breast milk.
	Carbamazepine (Tegretol)	D/L2	Avoid in pregnancy. Compatible with lactation. Monitor neonate for toxicity.
	Valproate (Depakote)	D/L2	Avoid in pregnancy. Compatible with lactation. Monitor neonate for toxicity.
Anticonvulsants	Gabapentin (Neurontin)	C/NA	Avoid in pregnancy and lactation.
	Lamotrigine (Lamictal)	C/L3	Compatible with pregnancy. Adjust doses in TM2–3. Compatible with lactation with monitoring of neonate due to high excretion in breast milk.
	Topiramate (Topamax)	D/NA	—
Atypical/typical antipsychotics	Lurasidone (Latuda)	B/NA	No known adverse effects in pregnancy. Level of excretion in breast milk unknown.
	Aripiprazole (Abilify)	C/L3	No known adverse effects in pregnancy. Level of excretion in breast milk unknown.
	Risperidone (Risperdal)	C/L3	No known adverse effects in pregnancy. Level of excretion in breast milk unknown.
	Quetiapine (Seroquel)	C/L4	Lowest placental concentration of atypicals. Low excretion in breast milk.
	Olanzapine (Zyprexa)	C/L2	Risk in pregnancy for LGA of fetus. Low excretion in breast milk.
	Ziprasidone (Geodon)	C/L4	No known adverse effects in pregnancy. Level of excretion in breast milk unknown.
	Haloperidol (Haldol)	C/L2	No known adverse effects in pregnancy. Compatible with lactation.
	Chlorpromazine (Thorazine)	C/L3	No known adverse effects in pregnancy and lactation.
	Trifluoperazine (Stelazine)	C/NA	No known adverse effects in pregnancy and lactation.
	Clozapine (Clozaril)	C/L3	Avoid in pregnancy and lactation.

Other Frequently Used Psychiatric Medications During Pregnancy

Antidepressants	Bupropion (Wellbutrin)	C/L3	Compatible with pregnancy and lactation.
SSRIs	Mirtazapine (Remeron)	C/L3	Compatible with pregnancy and lactation.
SNRIs	Trazodone	C/L3	Compatible with pregnancy and lactation.
	Fluoxetine (Prozac)	C/L2-3	Compatible with pregnancy and lactation
	Paroxetine (Paxil)	D/L2	In TM1, increase in risk for cardiac abnormalities but low absolute risk overall.
	Fluvoxamine (Luvox)	C/L2	Compatible with pregnancy and lactation.
	Citalopram (Celexa)	C/L3	Compatible with pregnancy and lactation.
	Escitalopram (Lexapro)	C/L3	Compatible with pregnancy and lactation.
	Venlafaxine (Effexor)	C/L3	Compatible with pregnancy and lactation.
	Duloxetine (Cymbalta)	C/NA	No known adverse effects in pregnancy and lactation.
	Desvenlafaxine (Pristiq)	C/NA	No known adverse effects in pregnancy and lactation.
Benzodiazepines	Clonazepam (Klonopin)	D/L3	Compatible in low doses with pregnancy and lactation.
	Lorazepam (Ativan)	D/L3	Compatible in low doses with pregnancy and lactation.
	Alprazolam (Xanax)	D/L3	Avoid if possible.
	Temazepam (Restoril)	X/L3	Avoid.
	Sonata (Zaleplon)	C/L3	No known adverse effects in pregnancy and lactation.
	Lunesta (Eszopiclone)	C/NA	No known adverse effects in pregnancy and lactation.
	Ambien (Zolpidem)	C/L3	Compatible with pregnancy and lactation.
	Chloral hydrate	NA	
	Hydroxyzine	NA	

Abbreviations: - D/C, discontinue; LGA, low for gestational age; NA, unknown; M1,2,3 = trimester 1,2,3.

was also added: L1, L2, L3, and L4 (see **Table 1**). Although the intention was noble, the classification system creates difficulties. Some of the difficulties with the current classifications are (1) it generates the misperception that the letters reflect a scale of increasing risk when actually they reflect different risk/benefit balances; (2) the categories do not distinguish between animal and human studies; (3) the categories do not distinguish between the types and severities of the various toxicities; (4) despite more safety data becoming available, the classifications remained static; and (5) commonly, patients and clinicians abruptly discontinue medications based on the classification, which leads to worse pregnancy outcomes. (Only 1 psychotropic has had its classification changed. Bupropion received a new indication for smoking cessation in 1997, leading to a change from category B to C; however, this was based on a new indication not on new data.)

The teratogenic risk categories have remained under revision since 2008. It would eliminate the current categories and instead provide a more clinically relevant framework to manage teratogenic risk and would follow the Motherisk Program model in Canada. The new framework will be based on intrinsic factors, such as scientific evidence in animal and human models, and extrinsic factors, such as clinical conditions and context of care, and provide updated discussions of current data. It will have 3 sections: (1) risk summary, (2) clinical considerations, and (3) therapeutic alternatives and data summary. At this point, however, the old classification system is still in place and provides little guidance for prescribing, which leads to treatment errors by clinicians who have little experience with the perinatal population. Therefore, although it may be helpful to know the classifications of these medications, treatment decisions should be clearly focused on the clinical presentation.

Discussion of Specific Medications and Risks

Pharmacokinetic changes in pregnancy

Pregnancy leads to many pharmacokinetic changes in the body. Understanding these changes is crucial to effectively and safely treat many medical conditions throughout pregnancy. Blood volume gradually increases to a peak increase of 40% to 50% by 32 weeks' gestation.[21,22] This is thought a protective mechanism to prevent hemodynamic instability on delivery; however, this leads to an increase in the volume of distribution of hydrophilic medications, requiring larger doses of such drugs.[21] Serum albumin concentration decreases, which affects medications that are highly protein bound.[21,22] These medications would have significantly higher amounts of unbound drug, requiring a dosage reduction during pregnancy.[21] Afferent and efferent arterioles dilate during pregnancy, leading to a 50% increase in renal blood flow and clearance.[21,22] Increasing renal clearance also increases the elimination rate of drugs that are cleared by the kidneys, producing subtherapeutic concentrations.[21,22] Sodium and water retention is also increased, producing a dilutional effect on plasma sodium concentrations as well as a decrease in peak hydrophilic drug serum concentrations.[21] The progesterone increase during pregnancy causes delayed gastric emptying, which leads to a lower peak concentration as well as longer time to peak concentration of oral medications.[21,22] The metabolism of medications may also be altered in pregnancy.[21,22] Phase I metabolism is affected by alteration of several cytochrome (CYP)450 enzymes.[22] CYP3A4 activity is increased during pregnancy, often requiring dose adjustments in medications metabolized by the enzyme.[21,22] CYP1A2 activity is reduced by 60% to 75%; CYP2C19 activity is reduced by approximately 50%.[22] CYP2D6 is often induced during pregnancy, but the degree of alteration varies on the allele form present.[21,22]

Phase II metabolism is also affected, including urine diphosphate–glucuronyltransferase (UGT) induction.[21,22]

At delivery, plasma volume drops dramatically, predisposing women to toxicity if dosages had been increased throughout pregnancy.[22] Renal clearance and hepatic metabolism return to preconception levels over the course of 1 to 2 weeks.[22–26]

Lamotrigine

Lamotrigine is one of the most widely used mood stabilizers and is one of the most studied among newer agents.[22,24,25,27–29] The alteration of pharmacokinetics in pregnancy has a great impact on women who are on lamotrigine.[22,25,27] Lamotrigine is metabolized by glucuronidation via the UGT pathway in the liver, which is induced during pregnancy.[22,24,25,27,30,31] This induction causes the blood concentration of lamotrigine to be substantially reduced.[22,24,25,27,30] This increase in clearance occurs at pregnancy onset and continues to progress throughout the duration of pregnancy, with clearance increased as much as 330% during the third trimester.[22–25,27] Clearance returns to preconception levels rapidly after delivery, starting within days after delivery, and is complete within 2 to 3 weeks.[22–25,27] The implications of this alteration in clearance could mean some women may not be adequately treated, putting them at an even higher risk for relapse.[31] When used for the treatment of epilepsy, several reports have demonstrated the need to increase lamotrigine doses throughout pregnancy to continue the clinical benefit (absence of seizures), and a more recent observational trial suggested that the same is true when used for bipolar treatment.[25,27,31] Of the 8 women in this trial, 3 required dose increases to continue the clinical benefit, which also suggests that the decreasing concentration of lamotrigine during pregnancy is associated with an increase in symptoms.[31] Although therapeutic drug monitoring for lamotrigine is not standard practice outside of pregnancy, it may be prudent to get blood concentration levels before conception to provide a patient-specific target to aide dose adjustments throughout a pregnancy.[23,27] The American Academy of Neurology supports monthly monitoring of concentrations and consequent dose adjustment during the course of a pregnancy to prevent relapse or postpartum psychosis.[27] This should be followed by rapid de-escalation of the dose back to preconception levels after delivery to prevent toxicity.[23,27,28,31,32] Clinical manifestations of toxicity include blurred vision, ataxia, slurred speech, dizziness, nausea, and malaise.[31,32]

Currently, it is unclear if lamotrigine exposure during pregnancy has an increased risk of major congenital malformations above background rates.[33] The overall risk of major congenital malformations with lamotrigine monotherapy is estimated to be 2% to 3%.[30,33–36] A few reports have suggested a potential increased risk of oral clefts, but other reports and multiple national registries (including 1 from Denmark with more than 830,000 live births) have found no increased risk of major birth defects, including oral clefts.[28–30,32,33,36] Some investigators have also suggested higher rates of major congenital malformations at higher doses (typically more than 200 mg/d), but most reports have not demonstrated a dose-related effect.[23,33,36] Congenital malformation rates have been shown lower with lamotrigine than with valproate and slightly lower than with carbamazepine; however, the rates are significantly higher when lamotrigine is used in combination with valproate compared with lamotrigine monotherapy (10.8% compared with 2.8%).[24,30,33,36] No evidence has suggested an increase in adaptive, emotional, or behavioral functioning or increases in neurodevelopmental disorder diagnoses.[33] Because of the extensive evidence that suggests safety during pregnancy, lamotrigine seems among the safest choices for bipolar disorder management during pregnancy.[33] It is FDA pregnancy category C.[37]

Lamotrigine use during lactation is generally considered acceptable; however, the drug is excreted in breast milk, and infant levels can be up to 50% of the maternal concentration.[28,32] Caution is advised when using high doses of lamotrigine in nursing women as well as in those with small or preterm infants.[32] Infants should be monitored for toxicity, because 1 case report of apnea has been reported.[28]

Clinical pearls
- Lamotrigine clearance is dramatically increased throughout the course of pregnancy. Clearance returns to normal rapidly after delivery.
- Drug concentrations should be monitored closely during pregnancy to ensure continued clinical benefit, and the dosage should be adjusted accordingly. Dosage should be reduced after delivery to prevent toxicity.
- Evidence supports the use of lamotrigine during pregnancy, with most data suggesting no increased risk of congenital malformations.

Valproate

Valproate has demonstrated an increased risk of major congenital malformations and birth defects when used during pregnancy, particularly during the first trimester.[28,33,36] The overall incidence of major congenital malformations is as high as 11%.[30,33,36] Valproate exposure has shown to increase in neural tube defects, spina bifida, craniofacial abnormalities, hypospadias, cardiac defects, and limb defects, and this is a dose-dependent effect (more malformations over 1000 mg/d).[28,30,33,35,36] Folic acid supplementation is recommended starting before conception and throughout pregnancy in hopes of reducing neural tube defects.[28,35,38,39] Conflicting evidence exists regarding this protective benefit, but supplementation is still recommended.[35,38] In 2011, the FDA released a Drug Safety Communication reporting that children exposed to valproate in utero are at increased risk for lower cognitive test scores compared with children exposed to other antiepileptic drugs.[40] Studies have also shown worse neuromotor functioning, worse adaptive and emotional/behavioral functioning, and an increase in autism and autism spectrum disorders in children exposed to valproate in utero.[28,33] Because of the numerous risks associated with use, valproate is FDA pregnancy category D when used for any indication outside of migraine prophylaxis, in which case it is category X (risks clearly outweigh the benefit for this indication).[41]

Valproate is a highly protein-bound drug, and its efficacy is due to the unbound drug that crosses the blood-brain barrier.[22] Clearance of valproate may increase by the end of the third trimester, which can result in reduced serum concentrations.[22] It is has been suggested, however, that the unbound drug concentration remains unaffected.[22] Valproate protein binding decreases during pregnancy, which could explain why free levels may remain unchanged.[22] If a decision is made to use valproate in pregnancy, consider monitoring both free and total valproate levels.[22]

Valproate is excreted into breast milk in small amounts, but there have been case reports of infants having thrombocytopenia and anemia as a result of exposure.[34,36,42] Although most investigators consider valproate use compatible in lactation, the manufacturer recommends caution be used if a woman is breastfeeding while taking valproate.[28,33,41]

Clinical pearls
- Valproate should generally not be used during pregnancy due to well-documented dose-dependent teratogenic risks associated with use.
- Most commonly, valproate use during pregnancy is associated with neural tube defects and spina bifida.

- *Folate supplementation is recommended before conception and throughout pregnancy.*
- Valproate is generally considered compatible with lactation.

Carbamazepine

Carbamazepine exposure during pregnancy is not as teratogenic as valproate exposure.[33] The incidence of congenital malformations is noted to range from 2.2% to 6%.[30,33,35,36] Carbamazepine, like valproate, most commonly increases the risk of neural tube defects and spina bifida.[28,33,36,38] As with valproate, folate supplementation is recommended before conception and throughout pregnancy to minimize these risks, although there are not many data to support this recommendation.[28,30,33,35,38,39] Carbamazepine also has been shown to increase the risk of cardiac abnormalities, cleft palate and other craniofacial defects, and hypospadias.[28,30,33,36,38] Exposure in utero has been associated with higher rates of low birth weight, growth retardation, vitamin K deficiency, and coagulation abnormalities as well as lower Apgar scores.[28,33,35,39,43] The long-term risks of carbamazepine exposure in utero are not clear. One prospective study has demonstrated a dose-dependent effect of worse verbal performance in 3-year-old children who were exposed to carbamazepine during pregnancy; at 6 years of age, this difference was no longer detected.[33] The FDA has determined carbamazepine to be pregnancy category D.[37]

Clearance of carbamazepine may increase during pregnancy, although evidence is conflicting.[22] Some studies have suggested a decline in total carbamazepine concentration during the second and third trimesters, but other studies have found no significant change throughout pregnancy.[22] The total concentration of carbamazepine may decline, but it seems that the unbound concentration may not change.[22,25] If a decision is made to use carbamazepine during pregnancy, both free and total drug levels should be monitored.[22]

Excretion of carbamazepine into breast milk is low, and lactation is generally considered compatible with carbamazepine use.[28,33,34,42] Transient hepatic dysfunction and poor suckling have been reported in infants exposed to carbamazepine through breast milk, so caution should be used.[36,39,42]

Clinical pearls
- Carbamazepine is most commonly associated with neural tube defects and spina bifida, although at rates lower than seen with valproate.
- *Folate supplementation is recommended before conception and throughout pregnancy.*
- *Carbamazepine is generally considered compatible with lactation.*

Oxcarbazepine

Oxcarbazepine does not have much safety data regarding use in pregnancy.[41] Denmark's Medical Birth Registry reported that among 393 pregnancies exposed to oxcarbazepine during the first trimester, there were 11 birth defects (2.9%).[44] Once adjusted for exposure to older antiepileptics, they concluded there was no significant increase in birth defects with exposure to oxcarbazepine above background rates.[44] More evidence needs to be established to draw conclusions about the safety in pregnancy.[45] At this time, oxcarbazepine is labeled FDA pregnancy category C due to the unknown risks.[45]

The pharmacokinetic alteration of oxcarbazepine in pregnancy is better established.[25] Oxcarbazepine is cleared mainly via glucuronidation.[24,25] Lamotrigine is also cleared through this pathway, which is significantly altered during pregnancy.[25] Small studies have confirmed that, like lamotrigine, oxcarbazepine concentrations decrease during pregnancy.[24,25] The decline is not as great, however, as that of lamotrigine, only a 30% to 40% decline.[25] Clearance seems to return to the preconception rate quickly after delivery.[25]

Oxcarbazepine is excreted into breast milk in small amounts, but evidence is lacking regarding the safety.[45] One case report of a women who switched to oxcarbazepine on delivery and breastfeeding an infant reports no adverse effects to the child through the age of 5.[46] Further studies are needed to establish the safety and risks associated with lactation and oxcarbazepine use.

Clinical pearl

- The risks of oxcarbazepine use in pregnancy and lactation are largely unknown at this time.

Lithium

Lithium remains one of the most efficacious agents used to manage bipolar depression and mania.[47,48] Historically, it was thought that lithium carries a 400-fold increased risk of cardiac defects, including Ebstein anomaly, based on retrospective data through the International Register of Lithium Babies.[33,49] More recent data are conflicting regarding the risk of Ebstein anomaly and other congenital malformations. Observational data have suggested a lower risk for Ebstein anomaly, 0.05% to 0.1%, after exposure to lithium in the first trimester.[28,33–35,38,50,51] This is still an increase from the background rate of 0.005%.[28,33,35,51] In addition, a prospective, observational study of 183 women exposed to lithium during their pregnancy found no significant difference between lithium exposure and no exposure regarding the risk of congenital anomalies, including persistent cardiovascular anomalies.[52] When spontaneously resolving cardiovascular anomalies were included, however, the difference was significant.[52] Alternatively, 1 meta-analysis found no significant increase in the risk of congenital malformations, including Ebstein anomaly, after in utero exposure to lithium.[48] The investigators caution that the sample size was small, however, and larger studies are needed before conclusions can be drawn.[48] A decision to use lithium during pregnancy must consider the risks of untreated mood instability and the potential risks the medication poses to the fetus.[38,47,49] If possible, avoiding exposure until after the eighth week of gestation is ideal to avoid exposure during cardiac formation.[38,39,50] At this time, evidence supports the recommendation to obtain a fetal echocardiogram and level-2 ultrasound during the second trimester in women who received lithium during the first trimester.[28,33–36,39,47,51,52] The FDA has given lithium a pregnancy category D.[37]

Infants exposed to lithium in utero have a higher risk of being large for gestational age as well as an increased risk of prematurity; however, this could be due to the bipolar disorder itself.[33,35,51] Neonatal adverse effects after lithium exposure include polyhydramnios, nephrogenic diabetes insipidus, thyroid dysfunction, floppy infant syndrome, and arrhythmias.[28,33,34,36,39,47,50,51] Neonatal adaptation syndrome has also been reported.[33] Neonatal adaptation syndrome includes hypotonicity, muscle twitching, dyspnea, feeding difficulties, arrhythmias, poor suckling, and cyanosis.[33] This syndrome typically resolves in 1 to 2 weeks and is thought associated with higher maternal lithium concentrations, possibly neonatal toxicity.[33] Because of the potential risk for neonatal toxicity, some investigators suggest stopping or halving the dose of lithium 24 to 48 hours before a planned delivery or at the onset of labor of an unplanned delivery.[33,39] Twice-daily dosing of lithium at the lowest effective dose could also be considered to keep peak serum concentrations lower.[38,39,47] Lithium should be restarted after delivery, once stable.[33] At this time, no data suggest an increased risk of neurodevelopmental adverse effects, but data remain limited.[28,33,35,38,51]

Lithium is completely eliminated by the kidneys, and clearance is increased during pregnancy.[22,27,51] Like lamotrigine, this could lead to subtherapeutic levels and put women at risk for relapse.[22,27,36] Clearance returns to preconception levels rapidly on delivery, putting women at risk for toxicity in the postpartum period.[22,27,51] Vascular volume drops as much as 40% at delivery, which also increases women's risk of toxicity.[22,27] Holding lithium for 24 to 48 hours before delivery (as discussed previously) has also been suggested to reduce the risk of maternal toxicity.[22,27,28,36,39] Hydration should be maintained throughout delivery, and some women may require intravenous fluids, in particular those with extended labor.[22,28,34] Therapeutic drug monitoring is recommended monthly during pregnancy, weekly during the last month before delivery, and on admission for delivery.[27,34,47,51] The preconception lithium dose can be resumed on delivery with lithium levels checked every few days until normalized.[22,27,28,47]

Lithium is excreted in breast milk, and infant levels have been reported as high as 50% of the maternal level, with most investigators suggesting a range of 20% to 30%.[28,39,51,53] Adverse effects have been reported in infants exposed to lithium through breast milk, although serious events are rare.[36,51] Lethargy, hypothermia, hypotonia, cyanosis, and ECG abnormalities have been reported.[28,36,42,51] Dehydration increases an infant's risk for toxicity and adverse effects as well as the decreased clearance of a premature infant.[39,51] If a decision is made to breastfeed while the mother is taking lithium, frequent monitoring of lithium levels, thyroid function, and renal function is indicated.[28] In general, breastfeeding is not recommended for women taking lithium.[33,42,51]

Clinical pearls
- Lithium exposure during the first trimester increases the risk of fetal cardiac abnormalities. A fetal echocardiogram and level-2 ultrasound are recommended during the second trimester.
- To reduce the risk of toxicity in both mother and infant, lithium doses should be held or reduced around the time of delivery.
- Lithium use is typically not considered compatible with breastfeeding.

Atypical antipsychotics
Atypical (second-generation) antipsychotic use has increased in pregnancy; however, safety data remain limited.[33,54] The evidence currently suggests a low risk of major congenital malformations, with rates ranging from 0.9% to 2.9%.[33] Few reports have suggested an increased risk of cardiovascular defects, such as atrial or ventricular septal defects, but the majority of evidence has found no increased risk of congenital malformations with the atypical antipsychotics.[33,34,49,55,56] The most consistent adverse effect during pregnancy is the weight gain that is commonly associated with use.[28,33,55,56] This weight gain not only increases the risk of obesity, gestational diabetes, hypertension, and metabolic syndrome in the mother but also may increase the likelihood of the infant being large for gestational age compared with typical (first-generation) antipsychotics or placebo.[33,37,55,56] The FDA released a Drug Safety Communication[57] in February 2011 stating the potential risk of withdrawal symptoms and extrapyramidal signs after delivery in infants whose mothers were treated with atypical antipsychotics during the third trimester.[28,33,57] Withdrawal symptoms infants may demonstrate include abnormal muscle tone, tremor, agitation, difficulty breathing, and difficulty feeding.[57] The FDA also reinforces that patients

should not stop taking these medications if they become pregnant without talking to their physician, and they should not be stopped abruptly.[57]

Data are limited on the long-term outcomes of infants exposed to atypical antipsychotics in utero. One prospective controlled study suggests decreased neuromotor performance at 6 months of age after exposure to atypical antipsychotics compared with children exposed to antidepressants or no psychotropic medications.[33] Another study reports delayed development at 2 months of age, but this delay had resolved by 12 months.[28]

Most of the atypical antipsychotics carry an FDA pregnancy category C label with the exception of clozapine and lurasidone, both of which are category B.[37,58]

Atypical antipsychotics are excreted into breast milk in variable amounts.[28] Serum concentrations are typically considered low in the infant, but adverse effects have been reported.[28] The benefits versus risks of continuing an atypical antipsychotic should be evaluated when deciding to use the drug while breastfeeding. The smallest effective dose should be used, and infants should be monitored closely.[28]

Olanzapine Of the atypical antipsychotics, olanzapine is the most studied, and, as a result, some investigators suggest it could be used as a first-line therapy during pregnancy.[59] Animal studies using doses 7 times the maximum human doses suggested no teratogenicity.[55] Most human data have also failed to show an increased risk of birth defects.[36,55,59,60] The rates for spontaneous abortion, stillbirth, prematurity, and major malformations have been reported as consistent with background rates.[36,60] Few reports have suggested low birth weight with olanzapine use; however, a majority of data suggest an increased risk for weight that is large for gestational age.[33,36,60] Olanzapine has the most weight gain associated with use out of the atypical antipsychotic class, which could lead to these metabolic disturbances.[36,39] Olanzapine is excreted in breast milk, and infant doses have been reported to be 0.3% to 4% of the maternal dose.[39]

Quetiapine Most evidence on quetiapine is in the form of case reports and 1 review that included 36 exposures to quetiapine during pregnancy, and no adverse effects were reported.[33] In 1 case report, a woman used quetiapine during her pregnancy and then breastfed the infant with no adverse effects.[36] Animal studies have suggested no increased risk of malformations.[55] The manufacturer's international database, including outcomes for approximately 300 pregnancies, has reports of 14 malformations with no patterns; it is noted that 11 of these women were taking other medications or there was only limited information provided.[55] Quetiapine has the lowest placental transfer of the atypical antipsychotics; however, it has the greatest incidence of sedation, which could be an issue for women trying to be alert to care for their child after delivery.[39] If a woman is clinically stable on quetiapine prior to conceiving, continuing on therapy is a reasonable treatment strategy.[59] Quetiapine is excreted in breast milk, and infant doses have been reported to be 0.09% to 0.43% of the maternal dose.[39]

Lurasidone Currently, the safety data of lurasidone use in pregnancy is unknown; however, animal studies have not demonstrated a teratogenic effect.[33,58] Although lurasidone was not approved at the time and as a result not included in the 2011 FDA Drug Safety Communication, the risk for withdrawal symptoms and extrapyramidal signs after delivery also applies to infants exposed to lurasidone in utero.[58] The amount of drug excreted in breast milk is not known at this time, and breastfeeding is not recommended with use.[58]

Clinical pearls

- Atypical antipsychotics have not shown an increased risk of congenital malformations. The most common effect on infants is a higher likelihood of large weight for gestational age.
- Infants exposed to an atypical antipsychotic during gestation could have withdrawal symptoms or extrapyramidal signs after delivery.
- Breastfeeding is typically not recommended with use of an atypical antipsychotic.
- If a woman is clinically stable on an atypical antipsychotic, the benefits of mood control and risks of relapse and fetal effects must be evaluated if she becomes pregnant.

Electroconvulsive Therapy

Overall, electroconvulsive therapy (ECT) is considered one of the most effective treatments for both MDD and bipolar disorder, with 50% to 75% remission rates. The most recent systematic review of case studies of ECT in pregnancy concluded that contrary to the prior systematic review, ECT should remain an option of last resort for pregnant women.[61] This article looked at 67 studies, a total of 167 cases, and noted that in 29% of cases there were adverse fetal effects, such as fetal heart rate slowing, uterine contractions, and premature labor during a mean of 9.4 administered treatments, half of them in the second trimester. There was a fetal mortality rate of 7.1%. Given the changes in administration of ECT over time, there was no reliable monitoring of fetal effects during and after ECT treatments. This is in contrast to a previous systematic review of 57 reports, 336 cases from 1941 to 2007, which reported only 11 cases of adverse fetal effects and suggested it as a safe alternative to the adverse medication effects needed to treat bipolar disorder.[62]

Despite the uncertainty that ECT is as effective in bipolar depression as it is in unipolar depression, a meta-analysis in 2012 stated that ECT is nevertheless an important treatment consideration for women with bipolar depression during pregnancy due to the risks of switching to mania when using selective serotonin reuptake inhibitors (SSRIs) for depressive symptoms.[63] This article looked at 6 studies of 1105 patients, of whom 316 had ECT for bipolar depression and showed remission rates of 50.9% and 53.3% for unipolar versus bipolar depression. Bipolar patients required fewer ECT treatments. This is important information to consider because treatment of bipolar depression with antidepressants can lead to acute mania, which can be even more difficult to manage during pregnancy.

Psychotherapy

There are few studies evaluating the effectiveness of psychotherapy for treating bipolar disorder in pregnant patients. Richards and Payne[64] reviewed alternative treatments to medications, including psychotherapies, light box therapy, exercise, and nutritional/herbal supplements. They noted that many of these treatments have been validated in the use of bipolar illness or as augmentation strategies, but data in pregnant bipolar patients are limited to nonexistent. Bipolar-specific cognitive behavioral therapy, family-focused therapy, interpersonal and social rhythm therapy, group psychoeducation, and systematic care management have all shown efficacy as therapeutic approaches for managing bipolar depression or preventing relapses. For pregnant bipolar depressed women, several researchers have suggested that these evidence-supported psychotherapies are likely beneficial as adjuncts to pharmacotherapy in dealing with psychosocial stressors that are known to have disruptive effects on illness course and increase risk of relapse.[33,65] This may be especially important when dealing with disruption of sleep and wake schedules or daily social rhythms.[66]

CLINICAL GUIDELINES

First and foremost, the goal is to keep pregnant/postpartum women functioning at their best. This helps in all other realms with both maternal and neonatal outcomes (short and long term), with their other children, with their relationships, with their socio-economic state in being able to maintain a job if needed, and with prevention of child abuse and neglect.

Secondly, this often necessitates involvement of more support by a spouse/significant other and family than at other times in a patient's life. This may also be a time in a patient's life when psychiatric intervention increases a patient's feelings of shame, humiliation, and worry that the pregnancy will seem imperfect. Thoughtful attention to these issues by a clinician ultimately leads to better adherence and communication with patient and family around the treatment plans.

Third, it is important to appropriately contextualize patient concerns. Clinicians may explain that major and minor episodes of depression are common during pregnancy and the postpartum period for all women, occurring in approximately 10% to 20% of the general population. Therefore, what they are experiencing is something that is shared with many other patients. Furthermore, clinicians may also explain that helpful treatments are available and that prevention and contingency planning are also important.

Fourth, the time when a patient is in the preconception phase is an excellent opportunity to review and potentially reorganize the medication regimen to establish the highest benefit and lowest risk situation before the patient attempts conception.

Fifth, complete a careful and thoughtful initial assessment. Clinicians start with a detailed review of the history, symptoms, and medication trials, keeping in mind that an assessment for undiagnosed bipolar illness is critical. Clinicians should include a review of all additional exposures to the pregnancy (ie, other medications, alcohol use, cigarette use, other substance use, interpersonal partner violence, socioeconomic stressors, personal and family history of birth defects, and developmental syndromes). The review of all past medication trials should include doses and duration and benefits and adverse effects.

Finally, the treatment plan that results from the assessment may occur under either urgent or nonurgent clinical circumstances. In either case, involving the appropriate supportive individuals in a patient's life and nonpharmacologic interventions are critical.

SUMMARY

In summary, medication management of bipolar depression in pregnancy and lactation is best done by assessing each patient's and family's needs in detail (**Box 1**). Keeping pregnant patients as psychiatrically stable as possible is the most important principle for clinicians, in conjunction with assessing the various risks and benefits of the medications. Unfortunately, there is no 100% risk-free situation for patients with psychiatric illness because both illness and medications present potential risks to mother and baby. This is often the most difficult and hard to accept reality for these patients, families, and clinicians. Clinicians serve these patients best by being as transparent as possible about the risk/benefit analysis of each patient's situation with the realization that ultimately the decisions are made by the patient and family.

> **Box 1**
> **Clinical pearls for pharmacologic treatment of perinatal bipolar depression**
>
> - Keep mothers stable—the best prevention of postpartum mood change is to maintain psychiatric stability during pregnancy and through delivery and the postpartum year.
> - In all evaluations, ask careful questions about hypomanic, manic, and depressive symptoms. More often patients seek help for depression not elevated mood.
> - Pregnancy is not the time to experiment with new medications—each new medication adds an exposure. If patient has a preconception period of time, consider medication changes at that time and contingency plans.
> - Discuss risk and benefits of both treatment and illness on patient, fetus, and family. The patient and family ultimately make the decision.
> - Be familiar with fetal development and windows of risk during pregnancy.
> - Treatment decisions during pregnancy must be made in conjunction with a treatment plan for the postpartum period and lactation.
> - Teratogenic classifications and lactation classifications should be considered but with the understanding that they provide incomplete information.
> - Consider the impact of illness on the patient's other children, spouse, and family.
> - Patients and families do best when they can make informed decisions based on comprehensive discussions with a clinician about risks and benefits.
> - Engage patient and family in postpartum planning around child care, patient self-care (including sleep), and lactation.
> - When using lithium, discontinue medication when contractions start to prevent maternal and fetal toxicity after delivery.
> - If a patient is on an antiepileptic drug before conception, consider use of atypical antipsychotics for the first trimester; if possible, return to the antiepileptic drug in second and third trimesters.
> - If lithium or paroxetine has been the most effective medication for a patient, consider changing to a lamotrigine or atypical antipsychotic for first trimester.
> - Obtain results of TM1 ultrasound to confirm normal fetal development.
> - Discuss patient/spouse/family religious beliefs and beliefs about abortion and miscarriage.

REFERENCES

1. Battle CL, Weinstock LM, Howard M. Clinical correlates of perinatal bipolar disorder in an interdisciplinary obstetrical hospital setting. J Affect Disord 2014;158: 97–100.
2. Clark CT, Sit DK, Driscoll K, et al. Does screeing with MDQ and EPDS improve identification of bipolar disorder in an obstetrical sample? Depress Anxiety 2015;32(7):518–26.
3. Merrill L, Mittal L, Nicoloro J, et al. Screening for bipolar disorder during pregnancy. Arch Womens Ment Health 2015;18(4):579–83.
4. Vega P, Barbeito S, Ruiz de Azúa S, et al. Bipolar disorder differences between genders: special considerations for women. Womens Health (Lond Engl) 2011; 7(6):663–74.
5. Viguera AC, Tondo L, Koukopoulos AE, et al. Episodes of mood disorders in 2,252 pregnancies and postpartum periods. Am J Psychiatry 2011;168(11): 1179–85.

6. Kessler RC, Chiu WT, Demler O, et al. Prevalence, severity, and comorbidity of 12-month DSM-IV disorders in the National Comorbidity Survey Replication. Arch Gen Psychiatry 2005;62(6):617–27 [Erratum appears in Arch Gen Psychiatry 2005].

7. World Heath Organization. The Global Burden of Disease: 2004 Update. Geneva, Switzerland: WHO Press; 2008.

8. Kawa I, Carter JD, Joyce PR, et al. Gender differences in bipolar disorder: age of onset, course, comorbidity, and symptom presentation. Bipolar Disord 2005;7(2): 119–25.

9. Nivoli AM, Pacchiarotti I, Rosa AR, et al. Gender differences in a cohort study of 604 bipolar patients: the role of predominant polarity. J Affect Disord 2011;133(3): 443–9.

10. Burt VK, Rasgon N. Special considerations in treating bipolar disorder in women. Bipolar Disord 2004;6(1):2–13.

11. Clark CT, Klein AM, Perel JM, et al. Lamotrigine dosing for pregnant patients with bipolar disorder. Am J Psychiatry 2013;170:1240–7.

12. Judd LL, Akiskal HS, Schettler PJ, et al. The comparative clinical phenotype and long term longitudinal episode course of bipolar I and II: a clinical spectrum or distinct disorders? J Affect Disord 2003;73(1–2):19–32.

13. Norhayati MN, Hazlina NH, Asrenee AR, et al. Magnitude and risk factors of post-partum symptoms: a literature review. J Affect Disord 2015;175:34–52.

14. Viguera AC, Whitfield T, Baldessarini RJ, et al. Risk of recurrence in women with bipolar disorder during pregnancy: prospective study of mood stabilizer discontinuation. Am J Psychiatry 2007;164(12):1817–24.

15. Bloch M, Rotenberg N, Koren D, et al. Risk factors for early postpartum depressive symptoms. Gen Hosp Psychiatry 2006;28(1):3–8.

16. Di Florio A, Forty L, Gordon-Smith K, et al. Perinatal episodes across the mood disorder spectrum. JAMA Psychiatry 2013;70(2):168–75.

17. Viguera AC, Nonacs R, Cohen LS, et al. Risk of recurrence of bipolar disorder in pregnant and nonpregnant women after discontinuing lithium maintenance. Am J Psychiatry 2000;157(2):179–84.

18. Bodén R, Lundgren M, Brandt L, et al. Risks of adverse pregnancy and birth outcomes in women treated or not treated with mood stabilisers for bipolar disorder: population based cohort study. BMJ 2012;345:e7085.

19. Jablensky AV, Morgan V, Zubrick SR, et al. Pregnancy, delivery, and neonatal complications in a population cohort of women with schizophrenia and major affective disorders. Am J Psychiatry 2005;162(1):79–91.

20. Lee HC, Lin HC. Maternal bipolar disorder increased low birthweight and preterm births: a nationwide population-based study. J Affect Disord 2010;121(1–2): 100–5.

21. Costantine MM. Physiologic and pharmacokinetic changes in pregnancy. Front Pharmacol 2014;5:65.

22. Deligiannidis KM, Byatt N, Freeman MP. Pharmacotherapy for mood disorders in pregnancy: a review of pharmacokinetic changes and clinical recommendations for therapeutic drug monitoring. J Clin Psychopharmacol 2014;34:244–55.

23. Adab N. Therapeutic monitoring of antiepileptic drugs during pregnancy and in the postpartum period: is it useful? CNS Drugs 2006;20:791–800.

24. Tomson T, Battino D. Pharmacokinetics and therapeutic drug monitoring of newer antiepileptic drugs during pregnancy and the puerperium. Clin Pharmacokinet 2007;46:209–19.

25. Tomson T, Landmark CJ, Battino D. Antiepileptic drug treatment in pregnancy: changes in drug disposition and their clinical implications. Epilepsia 2013;54:405–14.

26. Deligiannidis KM. Therapeutic drug monitoring in pregnant and postpartum women: recommendations for SSRIs, lamotrigine, and lithium. J Clin Psychiatry 2010;71:649–50.
27. Deligiannidis KM. Therapeutic drug monitoring in pregnant and postpartum women: recommendations for SSRIs, lamotrigine, and lithium. J Clin Psychiatry 2010;71:649–50.
28. Pearlstein T. Use of psychotropic medication during pregnancy and the postpartum period. Womens Health 2013;9:605–15.
29. Vajda FJ, Graham JE, Hitchcock AA, et al. Is lamotrigine a significant human teratogen? Observations from the Australian Pregnancy Register. Seizure 2010; 19:558–61.
30. Wlodarczyk BJ, Palacios AM, George TM, et al. Antiepileptic drugs and pregnancy outcomes. Am J Med Genet A 2012;158A:2071–90.
31. Clark CT, Klein AM, Perel JM, et al. Lamotrigine dosing for pregnant patients with bipolar disorder. Am J Psychiatry 2013;170:1240–7.
32. Vajda FJ, Dodd S, Horgan D. Lamotrigine in epilepsy, pregnancy, and psychiatry – a drug for all seasons? J Clin Neurosci 2013;20:13–6.
33. Epstein RA, Moore KM, Bobo WV. Treatment of bipolar disorders during pregnancy: maternal and fetal safety and challenges. Drug Healthc Patient Saf 2015;7:7–29.
34. Galbally M, Roberts M, Buist A. Mood stabilizers in pregnancy: a systematic review. Aust N Z J Psychiatry 2010;44:967–77.
35. Galbally M, Snellen M, Walker S, et al. Management of antipsychotic mood stabilizer medication in pregnancy: recommendations for antenatal care. Aust N Z J Psychiatry 2010;44:99–108.
36. Gentile S. Prophylactic treatment of bipolar disorder in pregnancy and breastfeeding: focus on emerging mood stabilizers. Bipolar Disord 2006;8:207–20.
37. Howland RH. Prescribing psychotropic medications during pregnancy and lactation: principles and guidelines. J Psychosoc Nurs Ment Health Serv 2009;47:19–23.
38. Eberhard-Gran M, Eskild A, Opjordsmoen S. Treating mood disorders during pregnancy: safety considerations. Drug Saf 2005;28:695–706.
39. Miller LJ, Ghadiali NY, Larusso EM, et al. Bipolar disorder in women. Health Care Women Int 2014;1–24.
40. FDA Drug Safety Communication. Children born to mothers who took valproate products while pregnant may have impaired cognitive development. Silver Spring (MD): US Food and Drug Administration; 2011.
41. Lexi-Drugs Online. Hudson (OH): Lexi-Comp, Inc; c1978-. Valproate Semisodium. 2015. Available at: https://online.lexi.com/crlsql/servlet/crlonline. Accessed March 31, 2015.
42. Eberhard-Gran M, Eskild A, Opjordsmoen S. Use of psychotropic medications in treating mood disorders during lactation: practical recommendations. CNS Drugs 2006;20:187–98.
43. Yonkers KA, Wisner KL, Stowe Z, et al. Management of bipolar disorder during pregnancy and the postpartum period. Am J Psychiatry 2004;161:608–20.
44. Mølgaard-Nielsen D, Hviid A. Newer-generation antiepileptic drugs and the risk of major birth defects. JAMA 2011;305:1996–2002.
45. Lexi-Drugs Online [Internet]. Hudson (OH): Lexi-Comp, Inc; c1978-. Oxcarbazepine. 2015. Available at: https://online.lexi.com/crlsql/servlet/crlonline. Accessed March 31, 2015.
46. Lutz UC, Wiatr G, Gaertner HJ, et al. Oxcarbazepine treatment during breastfeeding: a case report. J Clin Psychopharmacol 2007;27:730–2.

47. Bergink V, Kushner SA. Lithium during pregnancy. Am J Psychiatry 2014;171: 712–5.
48. McKnight RF, Adida M, Budge K, et al. Lithium toxicity profile: a systematic review and meta-analysis. Lancet 2012;379:721–8.
49. Jones I, Chandra PS, Dazzan P, et al. Bipolar disorder, affective psychosis, and schizophrenia in pregnancy and the post-partum period. Lancet 2014;384: 1789–99.
50. Matok I, Pupco A, Koren G. Drug exposure in pregnancy and heart defects. J Cardiovasc Pharmacol 2011;58:20–4.
51. Nielsen RE, Damkier P. Pharmacological treatment of unipolar depression during pregnancy and breast-feeding – a clinical overview. Nord J Psychiatry 2012;66: 159–66.
52. Diav-Citrin O, Shechtman S, Tahover E, et al. Pregnancy outcome following in utero exposure to lithium: a prospective, comparative, observational study. Am J Psychiatry 2014;171:785–94.
53. Moretti ME, Koren G, Verjee Z, et al. Monitoring lithium in breast milk: an individualized approach for breast-feeding mothers. Ther Drug Monit 2003;25:364–6.
54. Pearlstein T. Use of psychotropic medication during pregnancy and the post-partum period. Womens Health (Lond Engl) 2013;9:605–15.
55. Einarson A, Boskovic R. Use and safety of antipsychotic drugs during pregnancy. J Psychiatr Pract 2009;15:183–92.
56. McCauley-Elsom K, Gurvich C, Elsom SJ, et al. Antipsychotics in pregnancy. J Psychiatr Ment Health Nurs 2010;17:97–104.
57. FDA Drug Safety Communication. Antipsychotic drug labels updated on use during pregnancy and risk of abnormal muscle movements and withdrawal symptoms in newborns. Silver Spring (MD): US Food and Drug Administration; 2011.
58. Risbood V, Lee JR, Roche-Desilets J, et al. Lurasidone: an atypical antipsychotic for schizophrenia. Ann Pharmacother 2012;46:1033–46.
59. Ennis ZN, Damkier P. Pregnancy exposure to olanzapine, quetiapine, risperidone, aripiprazole and risk of congenital malformations. A systematic review. Basic Clin Pharmacol Toxicol 2015;116:315–20.
60. McCauley-Elsom K, Gurvich C, Elsom SJ, et al. Antipsychotics in pregnancy. J Psychiatr Ment Health Nurs 2010;17:97–104.
61. Leiknes KA, Cooke MJ, Jarosch-von Schweder L, et al. Electroconvulsive therapy during pregnancy: a systematic review of case studies. Arch Womens Ment Health 2015;18(1):1–39.
62. Anderson EL, Reti IM. ECT in pregnancy: a review of the literature from 1941 to 2007. Psychosom Med 2009;71(2):235–42.
63. Dierckx B, Heijnen WT, van den Broek WW, et al. Efficacy of electroconvulsive therapy in bipolar versus unipolar major depression: a meta-analysis. Bipolar Disord 2012;14(2):146–50.
64. Richards EM, Payne JL. The management of mood disorders in pregnancy: alternatives to antidepressants. CNS Spectr 2013;18(5):261–71.
65. Yonkers KA, Vigod S, Ross LE. Diagnosis, pathophysiology, and management of mood disorders in pregnant and postpartum women. Obstet Gynecol 2011; 117(4):961–77.
66. Harvey AG. Sleep and circadian rhythms in bipolar disorder: seeking synchrony, harmony, and regulation. Am J Psychiatry 2008;165(7):820–9.

Nutrition and Bipolar Depression

John L. Beyer, MD[a],*, Martha E. Payne, PhD, RD, MPH[b]

KEYWORDS

- Bipolar depression • Diet • Nutrition • Omega-3 fatty acids • N-acetylcysteine
- Vitamin D • Mediterranean diet

KEY POINTS

- Increasing research has identified the quality of one's diet as a potential major contributor to mood stability and expression. Mediterranean dietary patterns compared with Western dietary patterns may be supportive of good mental health in general and bipolar disorder specifically.
- Patients with bipolar disorder tend to have a poorer quality diet, with increased sugar, high fat, and carbohydrate intake. This may contribute to both poor physical health and mental health.
- Omega-3 fatty acids and N-acetylcysteine have been demonstrated to be helpful dietary supplements in the control of bipolar depressive symptoms.

INTRODUCTION

Nutritional psychiatry is an emerging discipline focused on the relationship between dietary patterns and mental health disorders.[1] Whereas the role of diet in physical health is well-acknowledged, the relationship between diet and mental health has received much less attention. The quality of diet is well known to be associated with many diseases, such as cardiovascular disease, type 2 diabetes, hypertension, and stroke. Therefore, changes that promote good dietary habits are commonly encouraged by health care providers to both prevent and treat these illnesses. However, the role of diet in mental health is much less known and with limited promotion among clinicians. Nevertheless, the impact that nutrition may have on the brain is self-evident. The brain operates at a very high metabolic rate, commanding much of the body's nutrient intake in order to support its structure as well as power its function. Nutritional psychiatry postulates that diet may contribute to either resilience or risk in mental illness.

[a] Duke University Medical Center, Box 3519 DUMC, Room 4082B, Yellow Zone, Duke South Clinics, Durham, NC 27710, USA; [b] Office of Research Development, Duke University School of Medicine, Davison Building/Green Zone, Suite 410, Durham, NC 27705, USA
* Corresponding author.
E-mail address: john.beyer@dm.duke.edu

Psychiatr Clin N Am 39 (2016) 75–86
http://dx.doi.org/10.1016/j.psc.2015.10.003
0193-953X/16/$ – see front matter © 2016 Elsevier Inc. All rights reserved.

Over the last decade, there have been an increasing number of well-designed studies that have demonstrated the association of a healthy diet with improvements in a variety of mental illnesses and symptoms, such as depression, anxiety, attention, and irritability.[2–9] Furthermore, their positive effect sizes suggest certain dietary interventions may be clinically relevant to patients, although as of yet, there are no available data regarding the therapeutic impact of dietary changes on existing mental illness.[10]

The effect of diet in major depressive disorders has recently been an area of more intense study. Two meta-analyses of diet and depression have supported the observation that a Mediterranean-style diet is associated with a protective effect on depression (as well as stroke and cognitive impairments), whereas a Western dietary pattern is associated with an increased likelihood for depression.[4,11] In another meta-analysis, Lai and colleagues[3] concluded that diets that emphasized fruit, vegetables, fish, and whole grains were associated with a reduced depression risk. These results suggest that what we eat may make a difference in how we think, or at least in how we feel.

Evaluation of the role nutrition and nutraceuticals may have in bipolar disorder has received only very limited research attention. At the turn of the century, the data that were available were often cobbled from secondary and experimental analyses of studies with other foci of attention, often confounding clear interpretation.[12] However, with the recent findings of the role that diet may play in depression and a new framework for understanding the relationship between nutrition and affective symptoms, there has been an increased focus on nutrition in bipolar disorder.

The purpose of this article is to review the recent research conducted on nutrition and bipolar disorder, with special emphasis on its depressive phase. Also discussed is the potential of nutritional interventions for bipolar depressions.

NUTRITION IN BIPOLAR DISORDER

In the past century, the food industry has undergone an enormous transformation, resulting in substantial increases of production, availability, advertising, and sale of food.[12] These changes have caused profound shifts in the composition of diets globally, which in turn, has contributed to the increased burden of diseases (such as cardiovascular disease, stroke, and hypertension) during the latter part of the 20th century.[13,14] As noted above, the Western diet has come under increased scrutiny for its role in these illnesses. A Western diet reflects a higher consumption of foods such as processed meats, pizza, chips, hamburgers, white bread, sugar, flavored drinks, and beer, a pattern that reflects high intakes of saturated fat, sodium, nitrites, and refined carbohydrates, including sugars. In health research, this dietary pattern is frequently compared with a Mediterranean diet, which emphasizes consumption of fruits, vegetables, fish, and whole grains, while limiting unhealthy fats.

Recent data from the SUN (Seguimiento Universidad de Navarra) Cohort study in Spain, an ongoing longitudinal study of 10,094 adults, demonstrated an inverse association between the level of adherence to a Mediterranean dietary pattern and the risk for depression.[7] Similarly, data from the Whitehall II cohort, a British based longitudinal study with 3486 participants, found an increased risk of self-reported depression after 5 years for those adhering more strongly to a Western-style diet pattern, and a reduced risk for those following a whole-foods diet pattern.[15] These findings have raised the question about diet and bipolar disorder as well, especially given the concern that many bipolar patients are at a higher risk of metabolic syndrome.

What kind of diets do patients with bipolar disorder typically have? There have been a few cross-sectional studies that have assessed the diets in small groups of bipolar patients. Jacka and colleagues[16] compared the diets of 23 women with bipolar disorder with 691 women without any history of depression. They found that bipolar patients had a diet with both higher energy intake and higher glycemic load than controls. Furthermore, the diet scores showed more consumption of the Western-style dietary pattern and lower scores for a traditional dietary pattern (vegetables, fruit, beef, lamb, fish, and whole-grain foods). Elmslie and colleagues[17] reviewed the previous 24-hour food consumption of 89 bipolar outpatients compared with 445 age- and sex-matched control subjects. They found that bipolar patients consumed more total carbohydrates, sucrose, nonalcoholic beverages, sweetened drinks, cakes, and sweets. Kilbourne and colleagues,[18] in their review of nutrition in veterans, evaluated lifestyle reports of 1945 veterans with bipolar disorder and compared that with 3086 veterans without diagnosed mental disorders. They did not find a difference in reported fruit and vegetable intake, but observed that this actually reflected the generally low level of intake in the general population.

What these studies underscore is that bipolar patients tend to consume an unhealthier diet, but it is unknown how diet and bipolar disorder may interact with each other. It is possible that poor diet quality may have a causative role in bipolar disorder. It is possible that poor diet quality represents a lifestyle factor associated with the illness. It is possible that poor diet quality may be caused by the treatments for the disease. It is possible that sweet and fatty foods are preferentially consumed by bipolar patients as a method of self-medication.[19] It is also possible that diet quality and bipolar disorder interact in more than one of these ways.

For example, in the analysis by Kilbourne and colleagues[18] of nutrition in veterans, behavioral factors in patients with bipolar disorder were also identified that would contribute to an unhealthy diet in anyone engaging in these behaviors. They noted that the bipolar group was much more likely to report eating only one meal a day, eating alone, or having difficulty in obtaining/cooking food. Poor nutrition access or limited diet options for bipolar patients may directly contribute to poor diet quality. The disease may be the cause of unhealthy lifestyle decisions.

Furthermore, in the diet review by Elmslie and colleagues,[17] the investigators hypothesized that the cause of the bipolar group's poor dietary patterns (increased consumption of sweets in the bipolar group) may be a medication-induced phenomena, because 87% of the sample were on psychotropic medications, which may significantly cause weight gain and metabolic syndrome. In other words, the treatment of the disease may be the cause of unhealthy diet patterns.

Lopresti and Jacka[19] noted that sugar may reduce stress-induced cortisol and therefore may be used excessively by bipolar patients, who tend to have more life stressors (or poorer coping skills). Furthermore, one of the primary symptoms of bipolar depression/mania is a change in appetite and weight, suggesting that the disease may induce the choice of unhealthy diet patterns.

Finally, others have suggested that diet may actually cause or worsen bipolar disease. Whereas in the past, this hypothesis was thought to be somewhat far-fetched, new understandings of bipolar disorder have caused us to rethink this possibility. Because of the nebulous association between diet and bipolar disease, further studies are required that control for the confounding variables in order that the role of diet in bipolar disorder may be better assessed.

THEORETIC FRAMEWORK FOR INTERACTION BETWEEN NUTRITION AND BIPOLAR DISORDER

Despite the increasing evidence of the role of diet in bipolar disorder, acceptance and translation to practice have often been minimized because of the lack of clear theoretic frameworks on which researchers can construct informed hypotheses and clinicians can integrate into effective interventions.[20] However, the increasing research on biological pathways that are dysregulated in patients with bipolar disorder has provided new insights into how nutrition may contribute to illness development. The improved understanding of inflammatory processes, immune functioning, and neuroprogression in bipolar patients has provided new hypotheses that challenge the understanding of mood disorder development and treatment. Lopresti and Jacka[19] conducted a review of several of these biological pathways that have shown dysregulation in bipolar disorder, and how diet may interact to induce or sustain these dysregulations. They include monoaminergic activity, inflammatory processes, oxidative stress, mitochondrial activity, and neuroprogression.

Monoaminergic Activity

For the past 50 years, the focus of mood disorder treatment, especially depressive episodes, has been on the monoaminergic neurotransmitters dopamine, serotonin, and norepinephrine. It is thought that alterations in neurotransmitter regulation and availability may cause a cascading effect on mood dysregulation. Animal studies have determined that high-fat diets may directly affect dopaminergic, noradrenergic, and serotonergic activity throughout the brain.[21–23] Furthermore, dysregulated dopaminergic signaling observed in obese rats that were fed a high-fat diet appeared to induce further craving for fatty foods.[24] Ketogenic diets that have been reported to help with depressive symptoms and bipolar II disorders[25] may exert their effect by increasing dopaminergic activity in the mesolimbic system.[26] Animal studies have also found that a high-fat diet decreased serotonin levels in the body[27] and prevented fluoxetine from effectively treating stress behaviors.[28] In humans, hypercaloric high-fat/high-sugar snacking has been noted to decrease serotonin transporters in the hypothalamus.[29] These findings suggest that unhealthy diets may not adequately support the neurotransmitters involved in mood regulation, or may even worsen mood symptoms.

Inflammatory Processes

For a detailed review of the potential role of inflammation in bipolar disorder, see Rosenblat JD, McIntyre RS: Bipolar Disorder and Inflammation, in this issue. This systemic inflammation may be caused by several identified processes, but 2 of these are nutritionally related: diet and vitamin D deficiency.[30] There has been consistent evidence that a Mediterranean diet and greater consumption of fruit/vegetables have been associated with reduced inflammation,[31–34] while a Western diet pattern has been associated with increased inflammation.[35] These relationships are further explored in the later discussion of omega-3 fatty acids.

Neuroplasticity and Neuroprogression

In the last decade, there has been a robust research interest in brain plasticity in mood disorders. Brain-derived neurotrophic factor (BDNF) is a neuropeptide that supports the growth and differentiation of neurons. Studies have shown that a Mediterranean diet was associated with increased levels of BDNF,[36] suggesting increased ability to nurture neurons. Numakawa and colleagues[37] have reviewed the interactions between diet and altered BDNF activity (noting also its association with inflammation). Animal studies have suggested that high-fat diets lower BDNF expression and decrease the quantity of newly generated cells in the hippocampus.[38,39] In their review of nutrition and neurogenesis, Zainuddin and Thuret[40] have found that caloric intake, meal frequency, and a diet composition of fats and sugars directly affected hippocampal development. More recently, Jacka and colleagues[41] found that subjects who maintained a Western dietary pattern over a 4-year period had a progression toward smaller left hippocampal volume than others on more healthy diets.

Oxidative Stress

A growing body of evidence has implicated oxidative stress and mitochondrial dysfunction in bipolar disorder. Mitochondria are responsible for energy generation and are extremely active in the brain, which is an oxygen-rich and highly energy-dependent organ. Impaired energy metabolism triggers pro-apoptotic signaling and oxidative damage; this in turn impedes mitochondrial DNA repair. These processes can potentiate each other, leading to a vicious cycle, whereby mitochondrial dysfunction leads to oxidative stress, which then leads to further mitochondrial damage and dysfunction. Studies have shown that diet may significantly affect mitochondrial functioning. A ketogenic diet enhances cellular metabolic and mitochondrial function, upregulates mitochondrial antioxidant status, and protects mitochondrial DNA from oxidant-induced damage.[42–44] In addition, a Mediterranean-style diet and elevated fish consumption have been associated with decreased markers for oxidative stress.[45–47]

BIPOLAR DEPRESSION AND NUTRITIONAL SUPPLEMENTS

The above examples of nutritional interactions with dysregulated biological pathways have provided better scientific hypotheses for understanding the potential diet/mood interactions. In their review of diet and depression, O'Neil and colleagues[10] noted that studies have consistently identified unhealthy dietary patterns as being associated with depression. They suggested that what is excluded from the diet may be as important as what is included. Although food is not the same as medication, it is increasingly evident that what one eats affects biological processes that in turn may affect mood. As of yet, the exact mechanisms in patients with bipolar disorder are not known, so consistent guidelines for dietary adjustments have not been codified. However, there are several specific examples that have been shown to be helpful in clinical practice.

Omega-3 Fatty Acids

One frequently mentioned dietary modification for use in bipolar disorder is the addition of omega-3 fatty acids. These polyunsaturated fats (PUFAs) have numerous health benefits, are significantly underrepresented in Western diets, and are thought to play a key role in promoting brain health. Omega-3 PUFA docosahexaenoic acid (DHA) and eicosapentaenoic acid (EPA), which are derived from marine sources (including fish and algae), are typically considered crucial for brain health and mental disorders.

The brain is primarily composed of lipids in a ratio of saturated fatty acids, monounsaturated fatty acids, and PUFAs. The principal PUFAs in the brain are the omega-6 fatty acid arachidonic acid (AA; $20{:}4n{-}6$) and the omega-3 fatty acid DHA ($22{:}6n{-}3$). AA and DHA are acetylated into the *sn*-2 position of membrane phospholipids of neurons. The enzyme phospholipase A_2 "activates" these 2 PUFAs by hydrolyzing the acyl ester bond. DHA and AA then exert opposing effects on the protein kinase C (PKC) signaling transduction pathway and the multiple downstream synaptic events regulated by PKC.[48] Eicosanoids (signaling molecules made by oxidation of 20-carbon fatty acids) derived from AA are pro-inflammatory, whereas docosanoids (signaling molecules made by oxygenation of 22-carbon essential fatty acids) derived from DHA are anti-inflammatory. Thus, if the membrane AA:DHA ratio is increased, there would be an increased inflammatory response detrimental to normal brain function.[49]

Emerging evidence has indicated that an inadequate intake of omega-3 PUFA may be associated with bipolar disorder. First, Noaghiul and Hibbeln[50] have noted in a multinational study that diets richer in the intake of fatty fish (foods high in omega-3 fatty acids) were associated with a lower lifetime prevalence rate of bipolar I, bipolar II, and bipolar spectrum disorders. Second, Evans and colleagues[51] found there was a reduced intake of omega-3 and omega-6 PUFA in the diets of patients with bipolar disorders. Third, Bly and colleagues[52] demonstrated that the diet of bipolar patients has a higher ratio of omega-6 to omega-3 PUFA (reflecting a Western dietary pattern). Fourth, animal studies have demonstrated that diets deficient in omega-3 PUFA alter monoamine systems in limbic structures.[53] Fifth, evidence from peripheral tissue fatty acid composition studies suggests that patients with bipolar disorder exhibit omega-3 PUFA insufficiency relative to normal controls.[54,55] Sixth, in brain autopsy studies of patients with bipolar disorder, DHA was significantly lower in the orbital frontal cortex (OFC) of bipolar patients relative to age-matched normal controls, and DHA composition was inversely correlated with elevations in AA and stearic acid conversion/metabolism.[49] (Of note, bipolar patients that committed suicide also exhibited selective deficits in OFC DHA composition, a finding that is consistent with studies in unipolar depression.) Seventh, mood stabilizers have been shown to specifically inhibit membrane turnover and downstream signaling of AA, but not DHA, suggesting that mood stabilizer activity may act in part by improving the ratio of AA:DHA activity.[56] Finally, systematic reviews of clinical trials using omega-3 fatty acids have consistently demonstrated a significant effect of omega-3 PUFA in ameliorating the depressive (but not manic) symptoms in bipolar disorder.[57–59]

As noted above, there are 2 principal types of omega-3 PUFA: DHA and EPA. Several reviews[60,61] have suggested that EPA, rather than DHA, is responsible for the beneficial effects of omega-3 PUFA in depressive disorders, and that supplements containing EPA greater than 60% were most effective against primary depression.[57] This finding is somewhat surprising given that DHA is a major structural component of neuronal membranes and EPA is present at relatively much lower levels. There are several possible explanations for this finding, including the fact that DHA is poorly incorporated into human brains and EPA may facilitate this. Other explanations include the anti-inflammatory effect of EPA-derived eicosanoids, its efficacy at reducing the inflammatory cytokines, tumor necrosis factor-α, interleukin (IL)-6, and IL-1b, and increasing N-acetyl-aspartate in the brain (suggesting a neuroprotective role).[57] However, methodological issues may also have biased the results in favor of EPA-containing prescriptions. The dose of EPA varied in each study, so the recommended dose in depressive disorders may be anywhere from 1.0 g to 10 g per day.[62]

The evidence for use of omega-3 PUFA in bipolar disorder suggests a positive effect in depression but not mania; however, the limited data available should give the clinician caution in their clinical expectations. Furthermore, current evidence only supports its use as an adjunctive treatment, not an alternative to standard psychopharmacologic interventions. On the positive side, omega-3 PUFAs do not appear to have any significant adverse effects and may be helpful for general health.[58]

N-acetylcysteine

As noted above, recent evidence has implicated the relevance of systemic inflammation and oxidative damage in bipolar disorder.[63] This evidence is supported by 5 prominent findings: (1) evidence of dysregulated oxidative defense in bipolar disorder, (2) effects of oxidative stress on cellular constituents (particularly lipids and mitochondrial DNA), (3) concordant structural evidence of neuroprogressive processes, (4) studies that have noted that bipolar treatments have significant influences on the oxidative processes, and (5) association studies of polymorphisms of key genes in the glutathione pathway.[64] Researchers therefore are interested in treatments that may target these pathways.

Glutathione is the principal endogenous antioxidant in the brain. It neutralizes reactive oxygen and nitrogen species and is responsible for maintaining the oxidative balance in the cell. Glutathione is vulnerable to depletion and substantially reduced in patients with bipolar disorder.[65] However, oral administration of glutathione is not adequate to replenish insufficiencies because it is rapidly hydrolyzed by first-pass mechanisms, and then only poorly crosses the blood-brain barrier. Therefore, researchers have focused on the use of N-acetylcysteine (NAC). NAC is a precursor to glutathione and provides L-cysteine, the rate-limiting factor in the glutathione synthesis pathway.[66] In addition, NAC has been shown to have anti-inflammatory properties that are linked to oxidative pathways.[65] Clinical trials in bipolar disorder have found NAC to significantly improve depressive symptoms and functional outcomes for patients during the maintenance phase of treatment over a 24-week period.[64,67,68] Secondary analyses also noted that NAC was helpful for bipolar patients with full depressive episodes and bipolar II patients.[68,69] The dose of NAC was either 500 mg or 1000 mg twice a day. Although these data support its use in improving depressive symptoms in maintenance treatment, trials are currently underway to assess its use as adjunctive therapy for acute bipolar depressive episodes.[70] The tolerability profile of NAC appears benign, but it should be noted that data on its safety and tolerability in long-term use are limited.

Vitamins

Vitamin D and folate are essential for good neuronal functioning and have been shown to be helpful in depression. Low levels of vitamin D have been associated with bipolar disorder; however, there have not been any studies looking at the efficacy of vitamin D treatment in bipolar disorder.

Folic acid and folate (converted into L-methylfolate in the body) have been increasingly used in depressive disorders. It is thought that folate may affect depression treatment by facilitating neurotransmitter production (modulating homocysteine and S-adenosyl methionine) and improving DNA repair and methylation.[71,72] However, evidence for its use in bipolar disorder is limited. Only one published study assessed the use of folic acid augmentation (200 µg) versus placebo in a small sample of bipolar depressed patients treated with lithium.[73] No significant difference was observed between the 2 groups in their depressive symptoms after 52 weeks. The negative finding of the folic acid study may be due to vitamin form, because folic acid, unlike naturally occurring folate, must first be reduced before it can cross the blood-brain barrier. Beneficial associations in depression studies have more often been found with natural folate and L-methylfolate rather than folic acid.[74]

Inositol, a vitaminlike substance found in many plants and animals, is a glucose isomer precursor of phosphatidyl inositol, an important second messenger system that is linked to neurotransmitter receptors.[75] Chengappa and colleagues[76] conducted a 6-week controlled trial using 12 g of inositol in 24 bipolar patients with depression. They found a significant reduction in depressive symptoms after 3 weeks, but this improvement was not maintained for the full 6 weeks. Another study of 5 to 20 g of inositol augmentation to mood stabilizers in 17 bipolar patients also found no significant improvement in mood outcomes.[77] However, possible efficacy was suggested by results from one of the STEP-BD substudies, a 16-week open-label augmentation of mood stabilizers with 1 of 3 compounds: lamotrigine, inositol, or risperidone, conducted in 66 treatment-resistant bipolar depressed subjects. All patients had demonstrated poor response to 12 weeks of a standard treatment or one of the randomized care pathways, or had a history of failure to respond to at least 2 antidepressants or an antidepressant plus mood stabilizer. The investigators found the rate of recovery was 23.8% with lamotrigine, 17.4% with inositol, and 4.6% with risperidone.[78] There is only limited information on the safety profile of inositol, so clinicians should use caution when considering its use.

SUMMARY

As with physical conditions, bipolar disorder is likely to be significantly impacted by diet and nutrition. Dietary patterns have been associated with bipolar disorder, including the potential protective effect of a Mediterranean diet. In addition, there is evidence in bipolar disorder of system inflammation and altered omega-3 fatty acid metabolism, both conditions that can be improved with dietary intervention.

Unfortunately, the evidence base examining the relationship between diet and bipolar disorder at this time is relatively thin. However, based on evidence for other brain disorders, including unipolar depression, there is optimism that nutritional alterations may have a definite role in the treatment of bipolar disorder as augmenters to pharmacotherapy. The most promising, in terms of both potential efficacy and safety profiles, are omega-3 PUFA, NAC, inositol, and L-methylfolate. These nutritional supplements have already been incorporated into some of the published bipolar depression treatment algorithms. The Canadian Network for Mood and Anxiety Treatment and the International Society for Bipolar Disorders bipolar depression guidelines[79] list augmentation with EPA and NAC among their novel or experimental treatment options, whereas the Texas Medication Algorithm Project for bipolar depression[80] lists inositol augmentation as a potential fifth step. Rakofsky and Dunlop[81] comment that given the limited evidence for these nutritional supplements, their placement at the end of these algorithms is appropriate.

However, more consideration should be given to the larger role of diet and nutrition in bipolar patients at the outset of treatment. Despite clear evidence of a link between nutrition and bipolar disorder, there remains a compelling reason to counsel bipolar patients to improve their diets. Individuals with bipolar disorder are at elevated risk of poor medical outcomes, including cardiovascular disease, diabetes, and metabolic syndrome, all conditions that may be prevented and ameliorated with dietary modification. Increasing intake of fruits, vegetables, nuts, and whole grains, while reducing consumption of saturated fat, processed meats, refined grains, and sugars, will improve a bipolar patient's overall health risk profile and has the potential to improve their psychiatric outcomes as well.

REFERENCES

1. Sarris J, Logan AC, Akbaraly TN, et al. International Society for Nutritional Psychiatry Research. Nutritional medicine as mainstream in psychiatry. Lancet Psychiatry 2015;2(3):271–4.
2. Jacka FN, Pasco JA, Mykletun A, et al. Diet quality in bipolar disorder in a population-based sample of women. J Affect Disord 2011;129(1–3):332–7.
3. Lai JS, Hiles S, Bisquera A, et al. A systematic review and meta-analysis of dietary patterns and depression in community-dwelling adults. Am J Clin Nutr 2014; 99:181–97.
4. Psaltopoulou T, Sergentanis TN, Panagiotakos DB, et al. Mediterranean diet, stroke, cognitive impairment, and depression: a meta-analysis. Ann Neurol 2013;74:580–91.

5. Rienks J, Dobson AJ, Mishra GD. Mediterranean dietary pattern and prevalence and incidence of depressive symptoms in mid-aged women: results from a large community-based prospective study. Eur J Clin Nutr 2013;67:75–82.
6. Rucklidge JJ, Frampton CM, Gorman B, et al. Vitamin-mineral treatment of attention-deficit hyperactivity disorder in adults: double-blind randomised placebo-controlled trial. Br J Psychiatry 2014;204:306–15.
7. Sánchez-Villgas A, Delgado-Rodríguez M, Alonso A, et al. Association of the Mediterranean dietary pattern with the incidence of depression: the Seguimiento Universidad de Navarra/University of Navarra follow-up (SUN) cohort. Arch Gen Psychiatry 2009;66:1090–8.
8. Skarupski KA, Tangney CC, Li H, et al. Mediterranean diet and depressive symptoms among older adults over time. J Nutr Health Aging 2013;17:441–5.
9. Jacka FN, Maes M, Pasco JA, et al. Nutrient intakes and the common mental disorders in women. Journal of affective disorders 2012;141(1):79–85.
10. O'Neil A, Berk M, Itsiopoulos C, et al. A randomised, controlled trial of a dietary intervention for adults with major depression (the "SMILES" trial): study protocol. BMC Psychiatry 2013;13:114.
11. Rahe C, Unrath M, Berger K. Dietary patterns and the risk of depression in adults: a systematic review of observational studies. Eur J Nutr 2014;53(4):997–1013.
12. Logan AC, Jacka FN. Nutritional psychiatry research: an emerging discipline and its intersection with global urbanization, environmental challenges and the evolutionary mismatch. J Physiol Anthropol 2014;33:22.
13. Popkin BM. Contemporary nutritional transition: determinants of diet and its impact on body composition. Proc Nutr Soc 2011;70:82–91.
14. Popkin BM, Adair LS, Ng SW. Global nutrition transition and the pandemic of obesity in developing countries. Nutr Rev 2012;70:3–21.
15. Akbaraly TN, Brunner EJ, Ferrie JE, et al. Dietary pattern and depressive symptoms in middle age. Br J Psychiatry 2009;195(5):408–13.
16. Jacka FN, Mykletun A, Berk M, et al. The association between habitual diet quality and the common mental disorders in community-dwelling adults: the Hordaland Health Study. Psychosom Med 2011;73:483–90.
17. Elmslie JL, Mann JI, Silverstone JT, et al. Determinants of overweight and obesity in patients with bipolar disorder. J Clin Psychiatry 2001;62(6):486–91.
18. Kilbourne AM, Rofey DL, McCarthy JF, et al. Nutrition and exercise behavior among patients with bipolar disorder. Bipolar Disord 2007;9(5):443–52.
19. Lopresti AL, Jacka FN. Diet and bipolar disorder: a review of its relationship and potential therapeutic mechanisms of action. J Altern Complement Med 2015;1–7.
20. Rucklidge JJ, Kaplan BJ, Mulder RT. What if nutrients could treat mental illness? Aust N Z J Psychiatry 2015;49(5):407–8.
21. Krishna S, Keralapurath MM, Lin Z, et al. Neurochemical and electrophysiological deficits in the ventral hippocampus and selective behavioral alterations caused by high-fat diet in female C57BL/6 mice. Neuroscience 2015;297:170–81.
22. Pritchett CE, Hajnal A. Obesogenic diets may differentially alter dopamine control of sucrose and fructose intake in rats. Physiol Behav 2011;104(1):111–6.
23. Wakabayashi C, Numakawa T, Ooshima Y, et al. Possible role of the dopamine D1 receptor in the sensorimotor gating deficits induced by high-fat diet. Psychopharmacology (Berl) 2015. [Epub ahead of print].
24. Corwin RL, Avena NM, Boggiano MM. Feeding and reward: perspectives from three rat models of binge eating. Physiol Behav 2011;104:87–97.
25. Phelps JR, Siemers SV, El-Mallakh RS. The ketogenic diet for type II bipolar disorder. Neurocase 2013;19(5):423–6.

26. Church WH, Adams RE, Wyss LS. Ketogenic diet alters dopaminergic activity in the mouse cortex. Neurosci Lett 2014;571:1–4.
27. Kim M, Bae S, Lim KM. Impact of high fat diet-induced obesity on the plasma levels of monoamine neurotransmitters in C57BL/6 mice. Biomol Ther (Seoul) 2013;21(6):476–80.
28. Isingrini E, Camus V, Le Guisquet AM, et al. Association between repeated unpredictable chronic mild stress (UCMS) procedures with a high fat diet: a model of fluoxetine resistance in mice. PLoS One 2010;5(4):e10404.
29. Koopman KE, Booij J, Fliers E, et al. Diet-induced changes in the lean brain: hypercaloric high-fat-high-sugar snacking decreases serotonin transporters in the human hypothalamic region. Mol Metab 2013;2(4):417–22.
30. Berk M, Williams LJ, Jacka FN, et al. So depression is an inflammatory disease, but where does the inflammation come from? BMC Med 2013;11:200.
31. Barbaresko J, Koch M, Schulze MB, et al. Dietary pattern analysis and biomarkers of low-grade inflammation: a systematic literature review. Nutr Rev 2013;71(8):511–27.
32. Chrysohoou C, Panagiotakos DB, Pitsavos C, et al. Adherence to the Mediterranean diet attenuates inflammation and coagulation process in healthy adults: the ATTICA Study. J Am Coll Cardiol 2004;44(1):152–8.
33. Holt EM, Steffen LM, Moran A, et al. Fruit and vegetable consumption and its relation to markers of inflammation and oxidative stress in adolescents. J Am Diet Assoc 2009;109(3):414–21.
34. Schwingshackl L, Hoffmann G. Monounsaturated fatty acids, olive oil and health status: a systematic review and meta-analysis of cohort studies. Lipids Health Dis 2014;13:154.
35. Nettleton JA, Steffen LM, Mayer-Davis EJ, et al. Dietary patterns are associated with biochemical markers of inflammation and endothelial activation in the Multi-Ethnic Study of Atherosclerosis (MESA). Am J Clin Nutr 2006;83(6):1369–79.
36. Sanchez-Villegas A, Verberne L, De Irala J, et al. Dietary fat intake and the risk of depression: the SUN Project. PloS one 2011;6(1):e16268.
37. Numakawa T, Richards M, Nakajima S, et al. The role of brain-derived neurotrophic factor in comorbid depression: possible linkage with steroid hormones, cytokines, and nutrition. Front Psychiatry 2014;5:136.
38. Kishi T, Hirooka Y, Nagayama T, et al. Calorie restriction improves cognitive decline via up-regulation of brain-derived neurotrophic factor: tropomyosin-related kinase B in hippocampus of obesity-induced hypertensive rats. Int Heart J 2015;56(1):110–5.
39. Liu X, Zhu Z, Kalyani M, et al. Effects of energy status and diet on Bdnf expression in the ventromedial hypothalamus of male and female rats. Physiol Behav 2014;130:99–107.
40. Zainuddin MS, Thuret S. Nutrition, adult hippocampal neurogenesis and mental health. Br Med Bull 2012;103(1):89–114.
41. Jacka FN, Cherbuin N, Anstey KJ, et al. Western diet is associated with a smaller hippocampus: a longitudinal investigation. BMC Med 2015;13(1):215.
42. Gano LB, Patel M, Rho JM. Ketogenic diets, mitochondria, and neurological diseases. J Lipid Res 2014;55(11):2211–28.
43. Jarrett SG, Milder JB, Liang LP, et al. The ketogenic diet increases mitochondrial glutathione levels. J Neurochem 2008;106(3):1044–51.
44. Liu Y, McNamara RK. Elevated delta-6 desaturase (FADS2) gene expression in the prefrontal cortex of patients with bipolar disorder. J Psychiatr Res 2011;45:269–72.

45. Fitó M, Guxens M, Corella D, et al, PREDIMED Study Investigators. Effect of a traditional Mediterranean diet on lipoprotein oxidation: a randomized controlled trial. Arch Intern Med 2007;167(11):1195–203.
46. Martínez-González MA, Salas-Salvadó J, Estruch R, et al, PREDIMED INVESTIGATORS. Benefits of the Mediterranean diet: insights from the PREDIMED Study. Prog Cardiovasc Dis 2015;58(1):50–60.
47. Mitjavila MT, Fandos M, Salas-Salvadó J, et al. The Mediterranean diet improves the systemic lipid and DNA oxidative damage in metabolic syndrome individuals. A randomized, controlled, trial. Clin Nutr 2013;32(2):172–8.
48. McNamara RK, Ostrander M, Abplanalp W, et al. Modulation of phosphoinositide-protein kinase C signal transduction by omega-3 fatty acids: implications for the pathophysiology and treatment of recurrent neuropsychiatric illness. Prostaglandins Leukot Essent Fatty Acids 2006;75(4–5):237–57.
49. McNamara RK, Jandacek R, Rider T, et al. Deficits in docosahexaenoic acid and associated elevations in the metabolism of arachidonic acid and saturated fatty acids in the postmortem orbitofrontal cortex of patients with bipolar disorder. Psychiatry Res 2008;160(3):285–99.
50. Noaghiul S, Hibbeln JR. Cross-national comparisons of seafood consumption and rates of bipolar disorders. Am J Psychiatry 2003;160:2222–7.
51. Evans SJ, Ringrose RN, Harrington GJ, et al. Dietary intake and plasma metabolomic analysis of polyunsaturated fatty acids in bipolar subjects reveal dysregulation of linoleic acid metabolism. J Psychiatr Res 2014;57:58–64.
52. Bly MJ, Taylor SF, Dalack G, et al. Metabolic syndrome in bipolar disorder and schizophrenia: dietary and lifestyle factors compared to the general population. Bipolar disorders 2014;16(3):277–88.
53. Chalon S. Omega-3 fatty acids and monoamine neurotransmission. Prostaglandins Leukot Essent Fatty Acids 2006;75(4–5):259–69.
54. Chiu CC, Huang SY, Su KP, et al. Polyunsaturated fatty acid deficit in patients with bipolar mania. Eur Neuropsychopharmacol 2003;13(2):99–103.
55. Ranjekar PK, Hinge A, Hegde MV, et al. Decreased antioxidant enzymes and membrane essential polyunsaturated fatty acids in schizophrenic and bipolar mood disorder patients. Psychiatry Res 2003;121(2):109–22.
56. Rapoport SI, Basselin M, Kim HW, et al. Bipolar disorder and mechanisms of action of mood stabilizers. Brain Res Rev 2009;61(2):185–209.
57. Hamdi A, Onaivi ES, Prasad C. A low protein-high carbohydrate diet decreases D2 dopamine receptor density in rat brain. Life Sci 1992;50(20):1529–34.
58. Montgomery P, Richardson AJ. Omega-3 fatty acids for bipolar disorder (review). Cochrane Database Syst Rev 2008;(2):CD005169.
59. Sarris J, Mischoulon D, Schweitzer I. Adjunctive nutraceuticals with standard pharmacotherapies in bipolar disorder: a systematic review of clinical trials. Bipolar Disord 2011;13(5–6):454–65.
60. Martins JG. EPA but not DHA appears to be responsible for the efficacy of omega-3 long chain polyunsaturated fatty acid supplementation in depression: evidence from a meta-analysis of randomized controlled trials. J Am Coll Nutr 2009;28(5):525–42.
61. Ross BM, Seguin J, Sieswerda LE. Omega-3 fatty acids as treatments for mental illness: which disorder and which fatty acid? Lipids Health Dis 2007;6:21.
62. Osher Y, Belmaker RH. Omega-3 fatty acids in depression: a review of three studies. CNS Neurosci Ther 2009;15(2):128–33.

63. Magalhaes PV, Dean OM, Bush AI, et al. Systemic illness moderates the impact of N-acetyl cysteine in bipolar disorder. Progress in neuro-psychopharmacology & biological psychiatry 2012;37(1):132–5.
64. Berk M, Dean OM, Cotton SM, et al. Maintenance N-acetyl cysteine treatment for bipolar disorder: a double-blind randomized placebo controlled trial. BMC Med 2012;10:91.
65. Dean O, Giorlando F, Berk M. N-acetylcysteine in psychiatry: current therapeutic evidence and potential mechanisms of action. J Psychiatry Neurosci 2011;36(2):78–86.
66. Berk M, Dean O, Cotton SM, et al. The efficacy of N-acetylcysteine as an adjunctive treatment in bipolar depression: an open label trial. J Affect Disord 2011; 135(1–3):389–94.
67. Berk M, Copolov DL, Dean O, et al. N-acetyl cysteine for depressive symptoms in bipolar disorder–a double-blind randomized placebo-controlled trial. Biol Psychiatry 2008;64(6):468–75.
68. Magalhães PV, Dean OM, Bush AI, et al. N-acetyl cysteine add-on treatment for bipolar II disorder: a subgroup analysis of a randomized placebo-controlled trial. J Affect Disord 2011;129(1–3):317–20.
69. Magalhães PV, Dean OM, Bush AI, et al. N-acetylcysteine for major depressive episodes in bipolar disorder. Rev Bras Psiquiatr 2011;33(4):374–8.
70. Dean OM, Turner A, Malhi GS, et al. Design and rationale of a 16-week adjunctive randomized placebo-controlled trial of mitochondrial agents for the treatment of bipolar depression. Rev Bras Psiquiatr 2015;37(1):3–12.
71. Crider KS, Yang TP, Berry RJ, et al. Folate and DNA methylation: a review of molecular mechanisms and the evidence for folate's role. Adv Nutr 2012;3(1):21–38.
72. Folstein M, Liu T, Peter I, et al. The homocysteine hypothesis of depression. Am J Psychiatry 2007;164(6):861–7.
73. Coppen A, Chaudhry S, Swade C. Folic acid enhances lithium prophylaxis. J Affect Disord 1986;10(1):9–13.
74. Payne ME, Jamerson BD, Potocky CF, et al. Natural food folate and late-life depression. J Nutr Elder 2009;28:348–58.
75. Qureshi NA, Al-Bedah AM. Mood disorders and complementary and alternative medicine: a literature review. Neuropsychiatr Dis Treat 2013;9:639–58.
76. Chengappa KN, Levine J, Gershon S, et al. Inositol as an add-on treatment for bipolar depression. Bipolar Disord 2000;2(1):47–55.
77. Eden Evins A, Demopulos C, Yovel I, et al. Inositol augmentation of lithium or valproate for bipolar depression. Bipolar Disord 2006;8(2):168–74.
78. Nierenberg AA, Ostacher MJ, Calabrese JR, et al. Treatment-resistant bipolar depression: a STEP-BD equipoise randomized effectiveness trial of antidepressant augmentation with lamotrigine, inositol, or risperidone. Am J Psychiatry 2006;163(2):210–6.
79. Yatham LN, Kennedy SH, Parikh SV, et al. Canadian Network for Mood and Anxiety Treatments (CANMAT) and International Society for Bipolar Disorders (ISBD) collaborative update of CANMAT guidelines for the management of patients with bipolar disorder: update 2013. Bipolar Disord 2013;15(1):1–44.
80. Crimson M, Argo T, Bendele S, et al. Texas medication algorithm project procedural manual: bipolar disorder algorithms. Austin (TX): The Texas Department of State Health Services; 2007.
81. Rakofsky JJ, Dunlop BW. Review of nutritional supplements for the treatment of bipolar depression. Depress Anxiety 2014;31(5):379–90.

The Influence of Trauma, Life Events, and Social Relationships on Bipolar Depression

Sheri L. Johnson, PhD[a],*, Amy K. Cuellar, PhD[b,c],
Anda Gershon, PhD[d]

KEYWORDS

- Bipolar disorder • Bipolar depression • Life events • Social support • Family
- Expressed emotion • Trauma • Early adversity

KEY POINTS

- Social environmental factors can predict a more severe course of bipolar depression.
- Childhood abuse is associated with a more severe illness course. Trauma exposure is associated with more severe chronic stress and greater reactivity to negative life events.
- Negative life events, social support, and sensitivity to interpersonal rejection, predict increases in depression.
- Family difficulties, and in particular family criticism, predicts more severe bipolar disorder.
- Clinicians should consider these social risk factors when establishing treatment plans for clients with bipolar depression.

The focus of this article is on the social environment as a predictor of bipolar depression. Although it has long been thought that bipolar disorder is largely a genetic disorder, a large literature indicates that psychosocial variables robustly influence the course of the disorder. This effect is particularly well documented for the course of bipolar depression.

Many clinicians argue that depression should be a central target in the treatment of bipolar disorder. Although the single diagnostic criterion for bipolar I disorder is at least 1 lifetime episode of mania, recurrent depressive episodes are a criterion for

Conflicts of Interest: The authors have no conflicts of interest to disclose.
[a] Department of Psychology, University of California Berkeley, 3210 Tolman Hall, MC 1650, Berkeley, CA 94720-1659, USA; [b] Michael E. DeBakey VA Medical Center, Houston, TX, USA; [c] Baylor College of Medicine, Menninger Department of Psychiatry and Behavioral Sciences, 1 Baylor Plaza, Houston, TX 77030, USA; [d] Department of Psychiatry and Behavioral Sciences, Stanford University, 401 Quarry Road, Stanford, CA 94305-5719, USA
* Corresponding author.
E-mail address: sljohnson@berkeley.edu

Psychiatr Clin N Am 39 (2016) 87–94
http://dx.doi.org/10.1016/j.psc.2015.09.003
0193-953X/16/$ – see front matter © 2016 Elsevier Inc. All rights reserved.

bipolar II disorder. Even within bipolar I disorder, in which depression is not a diagnostic criterion, depressive symptoms trigger more help seeking than do manic symptoms[1] and are related to suicide risk[2] and impaired functioning.[1]

People diagnosed with bipolar disorder vary greatly in the severity and frequency of depressive symptoms experienced. Many clinicians assume that all individuals with bipolar disorder experience episodes of depression (an assumption built into the name of the disorder), but as many as 20% to 33% of individuals with bipolar disorder report no lifetime episode of major depression (cf Ref.[3]). People who do experience depressive episodes vary a good deal in the course of depressive symptoms. Some people have only 1 or 2 episodes during their lifetimes, many have frequent recurrences, and perhaps the modal profile is chronic subsyndromal depressive symptoms. Among 146 patients with bipolar disorder followed for more than 12 years, depressive symptoms were present, on average, for about one-third of weeks.[4] Given this variability, a key question concerns the factors that predict the severity of depressive symptoms in bipolar disorder. Research findings suggest that the genetic vulnerability to mania does not explain the vulnerability to depressive symptoms within bipolar disorder,[5,6] and we argue that psychosocial risk factors are a critical part of this puzzle. This article reviews the socioenvironmental variables that have consistently been identified as predictors of bipolar depression: trauma, negative life events, deficits in social support, and problems in family relationships.

Differentiating the triggers for mania versus depression entails some methodological complications. Much of the research has been cross-sectional, and this work cannot disentangle the aftermath of episodes from factors that trigger symptoms. Manic episodes lead to occupational, social, and financial stress, and loss of self-confidence. Understanding whether the social adversities, in turn, intensify symptoms requires longitudinal research. This article therefore weights prospective research heavily where available.

EARLY ADVERSITY AND TRAUMA

In one recent study of euthymic persons diagnosed with bipolar I disorder, 61% reported a history of childhood abuse,[7] rates that are at least as high as those reported by individuals with unipolar depression.[8,9] Not only is childhood abuse far too common among those diagnosed with bipolar disorder, abuse is also associated with a more severe course of the disorder. In a comprehensive review that weighted 19 studies based on methodological rigor, childhood abuse (particularly physical abuse) was related to earlier onset, rapid cycling, psychosis, suicidality, impulsivity, aggression, and symptom severity, as well as more mood episodes, hospitalizations, and comorbidity in bipolar disorder.[10] In one study, childhood abuse was correlated with the severity of depressive, but not manic, symptoms within bipolar disorder.[7]

Some work has explored the mechanisms through which trauma increases symptoms. For patients with bipolar disorder, early adversity has been found to predict chronic stress[11] and reactivity to stressful life events later in life.[12] These changes in the levels and vulnerability to stress in adulthood may, in turn, shape symptoms.

However, most of the research in this domain has been cross sectional. In the 1 available prospective study of which we are aware, trauma history predicted greater chronic stressors across time, and those chronic stressors then predicted greater symptoms of depression, but not mania, within a bipolar I sample.[11]

NEGATIVE LIFE EVENTS DURING ADULTHOOD

Dozens of studies have considered life events and bipolar disorder.[13] Almost universally, these studies document that patients with bipolar disorder experience high rates of negative life events. In parallel, population-based studies indicate that people with bipolar disorder report high rates of adult victimization, with as many as a third of people with severe mental illness reporting that they were victims of violence within the 3 years before interview.[14]

Nonetheless, understanding the effects of life stress is complicated. Depression and related coping styles may contribute to the generation of stress in both unipolar[15] and bipolar disorder,[16] and so ruling out the influence of symptoms is an important goal. The best-validated approach for differentiating life events that may have triggered symptoms from those caused by symptoms is the Bedford College Life Event and Difficulty Schedule (LEDS[17]). LEDS assessment relies on a semistructured interview covering life events and their context. Raters who are unaware of the participant's subjective appraisal of the event then rate independence-the extent to which symptoms may have caused an event. Events triggered by symptoms are excluded from analyses. Raters also judge the severity of events, so that participants' mood state-related biases do not influence severity ratings. Life events may even be more common in unaffected family members of persons with bipolar disorder.[18] Again, this highlights the need for prospective research.

Prospective studies using the LEDS and related interviews have shown that severe, negative life events that are independent of symptoms predict increases in and duration of bipolar depression but not mania[19,20] (although see Ref.[21]). Bipolar depressive symptoms seem to be particularly related to events related to loss and danger.[22]

Negative life events were also found to predict the onset of mood disorders in a 5-year follow-up study of 140 offspring of parents with bipolar disorder, as assessed using the adolescent version of the LEDS.[23] Each negative life event increased risk of onset by approximately 10%. Parallel findings emerged when the investigators studied the onset of either first or recurrent episodes in a narrower 14-month period.[24] Because most (34 out of 38) onsets were depressive, the evidence supports negative life events as related to depression onset among people at risk for bipolar disorder.

Researchers have also considered whether the effects of negative life events vary across the life course. Despite long-held theory,[25] there is no consistent finding that life events are more powerful at predicting earlier episodes than later ones in bipolar disorder.[26] The most careful research has not provided much support for the idea that later episodes can be set in motion by less severe events.[27] Instead, older individuals with bipolar disorder, like those who are younger, seem to experience a very high rate of serious life events.[28]

Although research on bipolar depression has focused on the negativity of life events, other dimensions of events may also be important to consider. Sylvia and colleagues[29] found that life events that disrupted social rhythms were predictive of depressive symptoms and episodes in a sample of bipolar spectrum participants. However, other research suggested that life events that disrupted social rhythms were related to manic, but not depressive, episodes.[30] To date, findings are less clear concerning the role of life events that disrupt social rhythm as a contributor to depression severity (See McMahon K, Herr NR, Zerubavel N, et al: Psychotherapeutic Treatment of Bipolar Depression, in this issue).

LOW SOCIAL SUPPORT

As has been well documented in unipolar depression (cf Ref.[31]), social support seems to be an important predictor of illness severity and recurrence within bipolar disorder (cf Refs.[32,33]; for an exception see Ref.[34]). Social support deficits predict increases in depressive, but not in manic, symptoms over time.[35–39] People with bipolar disorder, on average, report being highly sensitive to interpersonal rejection, and those who report this sensitivity experience more depression over time.[40]

Research confirms that social support remains important in bipolar disorder across the life course, in that older (age ≥50 years) adults with bipolar disorder report lower perceptions of social support than controls, and they seem to have deficits in social support that are comparable with those of younger individuals diagnosed with bipolar disorder.[41] Social support also seems important in guiding older adults with bipolar disorder to seek treatment more quickly when symptoms do occur.[42]

Taken together, findings suggest that social support is an important prognostic indicator for depression within bipolar disorder. These findings seem to generalize across age groups.

Family Functioning

Family functioning is often poor for those with bipolar disorder.[43] In prospective research, family impairment has been shown to predict depressive more than manic symptoms among adults.[39,44,45] Nonetheless, overall social support (from a range of sources) has been found to be a more important predictor than the specific support obtained from family members.[39]

More specific indicators of family processes can powerfully predict the course of illness. One of the strongest predictors of course of illness is expressed emotion (EE), which is defined as criticism, hostility, and emotional overinvolvement of family members toward the patient with bipolar disorder.[46,47] Patients with bipolar disorder have a risk of relapse that is 2 to 3 times greater within 9 months if they live with a family member characterized by high EE.[48] Of the various facets of EE, criticism seems to most strongly predict outcome.[49,50] Two studies indicate that family criticism predicts depressive, but not manic, symptoms in bipolar disorder.[51,52]

In the past 10 years, there has been substantial growth in the literature examining the effect of family functioning on the outcome of youth with bipolar disorder. Poor family functioning is linked to suicidal ideation in youth with bipolar disorder.[53–55] Likewise, low levels of family cohesion and adaptability, and high levels of conflict, predicted symptoms of depression.[56]

Although the adult literature links poor family functioning primarily with bipolar depression more than mania, the adolescent literature is more mixed.[57–59] However, causal interpretations of family functioning on the course of adolescent bipolar disorder must be approached cautiously. One of the strongest predictors of risk of bipolar disorder is parental psychiatric disorder.[43] In addition, family conflict may arise as parents attempt to exert control over the manic symptoms they observe in their children.

In sum, EE and poor family functioning have clear deleterious impacts on the course of bipolar disorder. Although it seems that family functioning and EE specifically affect the course of bipolar depression among adults, family concerns may relate to both depression and mania among youth with bipolar disorder.

SUMMARY

Research findings indicate that early adversity, negative life events, low social support, EE, and poor family functioning may each help predict depression within bipolar disorder. These risk variables share extensive overlap with the social variables that have been shown to be important predictors of major depressive disorder. Given the strong parallels, psychosocial treatments developed for unipolar depression fare well in addressing bipolar depression.[60] Clinicians would do well to consider that reducing life stress, enhancing social relationships, and reducing family conflict may help improve the course of bipolar depression. Particularly given the chronicity of depressive symptoms, such treatment targets may have major repercussions for improving quality of life and well-being for persons with bipolar disorder.

Although not reviewed here, most of the psychosocial variables that predict unipolar and bipolar depression seem less predictive of mania. In longitudinal research, mania seems to be predicted by a set of variables that are related to positive affectivity, impulsivity, reward system activity, and sleep and schedule dysregulation.[61] Understanding and addressing mania may require targeting a host of other risk factors.

REFERENCES

1. Fagiolini A, Kupfer DJ, Masalehdan A, et al. Functional impairment in the remission phase of bipolar disorder. Bipolar Disord 2005;7(3):281–5.
2. Angst J, Cassano G. The mood spectrum: improving the diagnosis of bipolar disorder. Bipolar Disord 2005;7(Suppl 4):4–12.
3. Kessler RC, Rubinow DR, Holmes C, et al. The epidemiology of DSM-III-R bipolar I disorder in a general population survey. Psychol Med 1997;27(5):1079–89.
4. Judd LL, Akiskal HS, Schettler PJ, et al. The long-term natural history of the weekly symptomatic status of bipolar I disorder. Arch Gen Psychiatry 2002; 59(6):530–7.
5. Merikangas KR, Cui L, Heaton L, et al. Independence of familial transmission of mania and depression: results of the NIMH family study of affective spectrum disorders. Mol Psychiatry 2014;19(2):214–9.
6. McGuffin P, Rijsdijk F, Andrew M, et al. The heritability of bipolar affective disorder and the genetic relationship to unipolar depression. Arch Gen Psychiatry 2003; 60(5):497–502.
7. Erten E, Funda Uney A, Saatcioglu O, et al. Effects of childhood trauma and clinical features on determining quality of life in patients with bipolar I disorder. J Affect Disord 2014;162:107–13.
8. Levitan RD, Parikh SV, Lesage AK, et al. Major depression in individuals with a history of childhood physical or sexual abuse: relationship to neurovegetative features, mania, and gender. Am J Psychiatry 1998;155:1746–52.
9. Garno JL, Goldberg JF, Ramirez PM, et al. Impact of childhood abuse on the clinical course of bipolar disorder. Br J Psychiatry 2005;186:121–5.
10. Daruy-Filho L, Brietzke E, Lafer B, et al. Childhood maltreatment and clinical outcomes of bipolar disorder. Acta Psychiatr Scand 2011;124(6):427–34.
11. Gershon A, Johnson SL, Miller I. Chronic stressors and trauma: prospective influences on the course of bipolar disorder. Psychol Med 2013;43(12):2583–92.
12. Dienes KA, Hammen C, Henry RM, et al. The stress sensitization hypothesis: understanding the course of bipolar disorder. J Affect Disord 2006;95(1–3):43–9.
13. Johnson SL, Roberts JR. Life events and bipolar disorder: implications from biological theories. Psychol Bull 1995;117(3):434–49.
14. Choe JY, Teplin LA, Abram KM. Perpetration of violence, violent victimization, and severe mental illness: balancing public health concerns. Psychiatr Serv 2008; 59(2):153–64.

15. Hammen C. Generation of stress in the course of unipolar depression. J Abnorm Psychol 1991;100(4):555–61.
16. Koenders MA, Giltay EJ, Spijker AT, et al. Stressful life events in bipolar I and II disorder: cause or consequence of mood symptoms? J Affect Disord 2014;161:55–64.
17. Brown GW, Harris TO. The Bedford College life events and difficulty schedule: directory of contextual threat of events. London: Bedford College University of London; 1978.
18. El Kissi Y, Krir MW, Ben Nasr S, et al. Life events in bipolar patients: a comparative study with siblings and healthy controls. J Affect Disord 2013;151(1):378–83.
19. Johnson SL. Life events in bipolar disorder: towards more specific models. Clin Psychol Rev 2005;25(8):1008–27.
20. Johnson SL, Miller I. Negative life events and recovery from episodes of bipolar disorder. J Abnorm Psychol 1997;106(3):449–57.
21. Hosang GM, Korszun A, Jones L, et al. Adverse life event reporting and worst illness episodes in unipolar and bipolar affective disorders: measuring environmental risk for genetic research. Psychol Med 2010;40(11):1829–37.
22. Hosang GM, Korszun A, Jones L, et al. Life-event specificity: bipolar disorder compared with unipolar depression. Br J Psychiatry 2012;201(6):458–65.
23. Hillegers MH, Burger H, Wals M, et al. Impact of stressful life events, familial loading and their interaction on the onset of mood disorders: study in a high-risk cohort of adolescent offspring of parents with bipolar disorder. Br J Psychiatry 2004;185:97–101.
24. Wals M, Hillegers MH, Reichart CG, et al. Stressful life events and onset of mood disorders in children of bipolar parents during 14-month follow-up. J Affect Disord 2005;87(2–3):253–63.
25. Post RM. Transduction of psychosocial stress into the neurobiology of recurrent affective disorder. Am J Psychiatry 1992;149(8):999–1010.
26. Bender RE, Alloy LB. Life stress and kindling in bipolar disorder: review of the evidence and integration with emerging biopsychosocial theories. Clin Psychol Rev 2011;31(3):383–98.
27. Weiss RB, Stange JP, Boland EM, et al. Kindling of life stress in bipolar disorder: comparison of sensitization and autonomy models. J Abnorm Psychol 2015;124(1):4–16.
28. Beyer JL, Kuchibhatla M, Cassidy F, et al. Stressful life events in older bipolar patients. Int J Geriatr Psychiatry 2008;23(12):1271–5.
29. Sylvia LG, Alloy LB, Hafner JA, et al. Life events and social rhythms in bipolar spectrum disorders: a prospective study. Behav Ther 2009;40(2):131–41.
30. Malkoff-Schwartz S, Frank E, Anderson B, et al. Stressful life events and social rhythm disruption in the onset of manic and depressive bipolar episodes. Arch Gen Psychiatry 1998;55:702–7.
31. Brown GW, Andrews B. Social support and depression. In: Trumbull R, Appley MH, editors. Dynamics of stress: physiological, psychological, and social perspectives. New York: Plenum; 1986. p. 257–82.
32. O'Connell RA, Mayo JA, Eng LK, et al. Social support and long-term lithium outcome. Br J Psychiatry 1985;147:272–5.
33. Stefos G, Bauwens F, Staner L, et al. Psychosocial predictors of major affective recurrences in bipolar disorder: a 4-year longitudinal study of patients on prophylactic treatment. Acta Psychiatr Scand 1996;93(6):420–6.
34. Staner L, Tracy A, Dramaix M, et al. Clinical and psychosocial predictors of recurrence in recovered bipolar and unipolar depressives: a one-year controlled prospective study. Psychiatry Res 1997;69(1):39–51.

35. Cohen AN, Hammen C, Henry RM, et al. Effects of stress and social support on recurrence in bipolar disorder. J Affect Disord 2004;82(1):143–7.
36. Johnson SL, Winett CA, Meyer B, et al. Social support and the course of bipolar disorder. J Abnorm Psychol 1999;108:558–66.
37. Johnson L, Lundstrom O, Aberg-Wistedt A, et al. Social support in bipolar disorder: its relevance to remission and relapse. Bipolar Disord 2003;5(2):129–37.
38. Johnson SL, Meyer B, Winett C, et al. Social support and self-esteem predict changes in bipolar depression but not mania. J Affect Disord 2000;58(1):79–86.
39. Weinstock LM, Miller IW. Psychosocial predictors of mood symptoms one year after acute phase treatment of bipolar I disorder. Compr Psychiatry 2010;51(5):497–503.
40. Ng TH, Johnson SL. Rejection sensitivity is associated with quality of life, psychosocial outcome, and the course of depression in euthymic patients with bipolar I disorder. Cognit Ther Res 2013;37(6):1169–78.
41. Beyer JL, Kuchibhatla M, Looney C, et al. Social support in elderly patients with bipolar disorder. Bipolar Disord 2003;5(1):22–7.
42. Beyer JL, Greenberg RL, Marino P, et al. Social support in late life mania: GERI-BD. Int J Geriatr Psychiatry 2014;29(10):1028–32.
43. Chen YC, Kao CF, Lu MK, et al. The relationship of family characteristics and bipolar disorder using causal-pie models. Eur Psychiatry 2014;29(1):36–43.
44. Gitlin MJ, Swendsen J, Heller TL, et al. Relapse and impairment in bipolar disorder. Am J Psychiatry 1995;152(11):1635–40.
45. Townsend LD, Demeter CA, Youngstrom E, et al. Family conflict moderates response to pharmacological intervention in pediatric bipolar disorder. J Child Adolesc Psychopharmacol 2007;17(6):843–52.
46. Butzlaff RL, Hooley JM. Expressed emotion and psychiatric relapse: a meta-analysis. Arch Gen Psychiatry 1998;55:547–53.
47. Miklowitz DJ, Goldstein MJ, Nuechterlein KH, et al. Family factors and the course of bipolar affective disorder. Arch Gen Psychiatry 1988;45(3):225.
48. Barrowclough C, Hooley JM. Attributions and expressed emotion: a review. Clin Psychol Rev 2003;23(6):849–80.
49. Hooley JM, Rosen LR, Richters JE. Expressed emotion: toward clarification of a critical construct. In: Miller G, editor. The behavioral high-risk paradigm in psychopathology. New York: Springer; 1995. p. 88–120.
50. Rosenfarb IS, Miklowitz DJ, Goldstein MJ, et al. Family transactions and relapse in bipolar disorder. Fam Process 2001;40(1):5–14.
51. Kim EY, Miklowitz DJ. Expressed emotion as a predictor of outcome among bipolar patients undergoing family therapy. J Affect Disord 2004;82(3):343–52.
52. Yan LJ, Hammen C, Cohen AN, et al. Expressed emotion versus relationship quality variable in the prediction of recurrence in bipolar patients. J Affect Disord 2004;83:199–206.
53. Goldstein TR, Birmaher B, Axelson D, et al. Psychosocial functioning among bipolar youth. J Affect Disord 2009;114(1–3):174–83.
54. Weinstein SM, Van Meter A, Katz AC, et al. Cognitive and family correlates of current suicidal ideation in children with bipolar disorder. J Affect Disord 2015;173:15–21.
55. Ellis AJ, Portnoff LC, Axelson DA, et al. Parental expressed emotion and suicidal ideation in adolescents with bipolar disorder. Psychiatry Res 2014;216(2):213–6.
56. Sullivan AE, Judd CM, Axelson DA, et al. Family functioning and the course of adolescent bipolar disorder. Behav Ther 2012;43(4):837–47.
57. Geller B, Tillman R, Craney JL, et al. Four-year prospective outcome and natural history of mania in children with a prepubertal and early adolescent bipolar disorder phenotype. Arch Gen Psychiatry 2004;61(5):459–67.

58. Geller B, Craney JL, Bolhofner K, et al. Two-year prospective follow-up of children with a prepubertal and early adolescent bipolar disorder phenotype. Am J Psychiatry 2002;159(6):927–33.

59. Sullivan PF, Daly MJ, O'Donovan M. Genetic architectures of psychiatric disorders: the emerging picture and its implications. Nat Rev Genet 2012;13(8): 537–51.

60. Miklowitz DJ, Johnson SL. The psychopathology and treatment of bipolar disorder. Annu Rev Clin Psychol 2006;2:199–235.

61. Johnson SL, Cuellar AK, Peckham AD. Risk factors for bipolar disorder. In: Gotlib IH, Hammen C, editors. Handbook of depression. 3rd edition. New York: Guilford Press; 2014. p. 315–34.

Bipolar Depression and Cognitive Impairment
Shared Mechanisms and New Treatment Avenues

Colin A. Depp, PhD[a,b,*], Sheena Dev, BS[a,c,1], Lisa T. Eyler, PhD[a,b,1]

KEYWORDS

• Neuropsychology • Mood disorders • Aging • Brain function • Health behavior

KEY POINTS

- Depressive symptoms and cognitive impairment together account for most disability experienced by people with bipolar disorder.
- Bipolar depression and cognitive impairment seem to share neurobiological determinants, such as inflammation, as well as behavioral risks, such as sedentary lifestyles.
- Novel treatment avenues that may jointly target depression and cognitive impairment include pharmacologic agents and modification of health behavior.

INTRODUCTION

For many years, bipolar disorder (BD) was not believed to be associated with durable cognitive problems. A return to normal cognitive function was believed to be one of the main distinguishing features of BD compared with schizophrenia. However, over the past 15 years, scores of studies have accumulated to indicate that BD is associated with clinically significant cognitive impairments evident both during mood episodes and during clinically euthymic periods. Collectively, depressive symptoms and cognitive impairment account for most of the disability produced by BD. There remains a great need for efficacious treatments targeting either bipolar depression or cognitive dysfunction. Emerging research has shifted away from efforts to parse cognitive deficits from mood symptoms toward examining their shared neurobiological mechanisms, behavioral determinants, and treatment avenues.

Disclosures: None of the authors has any conflicts of interests to report.
Role of the Funding Source: The study was funded in part by the National Institute of Mental Health Grants MH100417 and MH100318.
[a] Department of Psychiatry, UC San Diego, 9500 Gilman Drive, La Jolla, CA 92093, USA; [b] Desert-Pacific Mental Illness Research, Education, and Clinical Center, VA San Diego Healthcare System, 3350 La Jolla Village Drive, San Diego, CA 92161, USA; [c] SDSU-UCSD Joint Doctoral Program, Clinical Psychology, San Diego, CA, USA
[1] Present address: 3350 La Jolla Village Drive, VMRF Building 13, San Diego, CA 92161.
* Corresponding author. UC San Diego, 9500 Gilman Drive (0664), La Jolla, CA 92093-0664.
E-mail address: cdepp@ucsd.edu

Psychiatr Clin N Am 39 (2016) 95–109
http://dx.doi.org/10.1016/j.psc.2015.09.004
0193-953X/16/$ – see front matter Published by Elsevier Inc.

PREVALENCE AND DISTRIBUTION OF COGNITIVE IMPAIRMENTS IN EUTHYMIC PATIENTS

The distribution of cognitive deficits in BD, as with most aspects of this illness, is heterogeneous and complex. Approximately 40% to 60% of patients with BD show clinically significant cognitive impairment.[1] Thus, although cognitive impairment may enact a marked impact on functioning at the population level in BD, global cognitive impairment is not evident in approximately half of patients. Within the BD spectrum, there is some evidence that risk of cognitive impairment varies by diagnostic subtype and clinical features. Some studies[2] have found that cognitive deficits are more prominent in patients with bipolar I versus bipolar II disorders, although this finding is not consistent.[3] A history of psychotic features, more common in bipolar I compared with bipolar II, is also associated with a greater likelihood of cognitive impairment.[4]

Some cognitive abilities seem more affected by BD. In meta-analyses that have examined cognitive performance in euthymic patients compared with performance in healthy control individuals,[5,6] deficits are apparent at medium to large effect sizes in the areas of verbal memory, executive function, processing speed, and sustained attention. In contrast, vocabulary, naming, and verbal fluency abilities are generally observed to be comparable with those of healthy comparators. A recent study by Burdick and colleagues[7] used cluster analysis to indicate that roughly 40% of patients showed normal cognition, 30% showed selective deficits in verbal memory, processing speed, attention, and social cognition yet with normal functioning, and 30% were globally cognitively and functionally impaired.

An increasing number of studies have investigated domains of cognition that extend beyond traditional neuropsychological foci, such as social cognitive abilities. In a recent meta-analysis in euthymic patients across a range of social cognition measures,[8] deficits were present in theory of mind and emotional reasoning tasks, whereas basic emotion recognition tasks were preserved.

COMPARISON OF COGNITIVE DEFICITS IN BIPOLAR DISORDER WITH THOSE IN OTHER PSYCHIATRIC ILLNESSES

Compared with schizophrenia, the neuropsychological deficits of BD seem to be less severe and more selective. The rate of global cognitive impairment in schizophrenia is 90%, and a meta-analysis of cognitive function comparing schizophrenia with BD[9] reported a mean difference between these disorders of about a half of a standard deviation, with individuals with BD performing better. Severity distinctions compared with unipolar depression are less clear and seem to vary by clinical state and medication status. For example, one study[10] indicated greater impairment in unmedicated unipolar depressed patients compared with patients with bipolar II disorder. Another longitudinal study[11] found evidence of increased dysfunction in patients with bipolar I after treatment of acute depression but similar cognitive test performance during acute depression, and, in another study,[12] similarities in brain activation between bipolar and unipolar acutely depressed patients were seen. Thus, the balance of evidence indicates that on a spectrum of cognitive impairment, BD is intermediate between unipolar depression and schizophrenia, particularly when comparing across mood disorders in euthymic states.

STUDIES OF THE SHORTER-TERM EFFECT OF BIPOLAR DEPRESSION ON COGNITIVE FUNCTION

Several studies have evaluated cognition in samples of patients with BD during the presence of active depressive symptoms versus euthymic or hypo/manic states.

There is considerable variability, with a meta-analysis[13] finding some evidence that bipolar depression was associated with poorer fluency and verbal learning. Additional work[14,15] found comparable performance in depressed versus euthymic patients, although others[16] have found depressed patients were more likely to show deficits in verbal recall and fine motor skills than euthymic patients. Over the short-term (1 year) in first-episode patients, a prospective study[17] found no association between recurrence of depression and change in cognitive functioning. Patients with a verbal memory deficit in this study were more at risk for mood relapse. Overall, there seems to be some exaggeration of specific deficits by depression, but the impact of the depressed state seems smaller than that associated with the presence of the bipolar diagnosis compared with healthy comparison individuals.

STUDIES OF THE LONG-TERM EFFECT OF BIPOLAR DEPRESSION ON COGNITIVE FUNCTION

Some investigators have recently proposed that BD may involve a progressive neurodegenerative decline in cognitive function and that BD is associated with neuroprogression.[18,19] Although there is some neurobiological evidence in favor of this deterioration in cognition hypothesis, the small number of longer-term follow-up studies (3–10 years) have failed to consistently support that cognitive abilities decline at a faster rate in patients with BD than in normal control individuals.

Nonetheless, a seminal review by Robinson and Ferrier[20] found some evidence that patients with a history of more hospitalizations, longer duration of illness, and more severe manic symptoms were more likely to show cognitive impairments. Little evidence suggested that more frequent or severe depressive episodes were associated with deteriorating trajectories of cognitive function in the context of BD. Of course, cross-sectional studies cannot confirm causal effects of mood symptoms on longer-term cognitive impairment, because patients with more severe courses of affective symptoms may also have more severe cognitive deficits. However, more generally, recent longitudinal research has suggested that depressive symptoms precede and predict memory decline in nondemented elderly adults, leaving open the possibility that depressive symptoms could contribute to declines in BD if measured longitudinally.[21]

Over the long-term, there is some suggestion that cumulative effects of mood episodes may foster cognitive deterioration. These life-course findings have led to discussion of stage models of BD in which earlier stages are associated with more episodic depression and latter stages with more cognitive impairment, disability, and persistent depression.[22]

IMPACT OF COGNITIVE IMPAIRMENT AND DEPRESSION ON PSYCHOSOCIAL FUNCTIONING

A sizable body of research has shown that cognitive ability is associated with psychosocial disability in BD. In a recent meta-analysis, the strength of this association was identical to that in a separate meta-analysis of studies examining the same question in schizophrenia.[23] This finding may indicate that even if the level of disability experienced by people with BD is lower than that experienced in schizophrenia, the average impact of cognitive impairment is comparable. An even larger body of literature, including the seminal prospective studies of Judd and colleagues,[24] has indicated that increases in bipolar depression even at the subsyndromal level account for a remarkable proportion of disability. Cognitive impairment and depression collectively produce most disability in this illness.

There are emerging data that suggest nuances in the combined impact of cognitive impairment and bipolar depression on psychosocial function. Bowie and colleagues[25] found that bipolar depression and cognitive ability were independently associated with occupational performance and interpersonal function, mediated through measures of capacity to perform these functional tasks. However, cognitive ability, but not depression, was associated with performance of instrumental activities of daily living. Over a 1-year period, Bonnin and colleagues[26] found that verbal memory deficits exacerbated the impact of subsyndromal depression on functional outcome. Cognitive impairment and depression likely amplify each other in producing disability, and the relative impact of each may differ by domain of disability. Depp and colleagues[27] found that cognitive impairment was associated with whether or not patients were engaged in competitive employment and depression was associated with the number of hours worked in those employed. The investigators speculated that cognitive impairment could be seen as rate limiting in the acquisition of employment, whereas depression was more relevant to producing disability in the comparatively less cognitively impaired patients who were employed.

Further understanding of the confluence of depression and cognitive ability may come from studies on self-assessment of performance. Emerging research[28] indicates that bipolar depression influences self-assessment of performance on objective cognitive and functional tasks and patients who evaluate their performance as poor are less likely to seek and attain functional milestones such as employment irrespective of their capacity to engage in such tasks. In this way, depression may exacerbate the impact of mild cognitive deficits on functioning by introducing self-defeating biases.

POTENTIAL PATHWAYS BETWEEN DEPRESSION AND COGNITIVE IMPAIRMENT

Research has pointed to at least 3 possible pathways between cognitive impairment and bipolar depression:

1. Sustained and recurrent mood symptoms may directly affect neurobiological pathways that diminish cognitive ability;
2. Mood symptoms may indirectly contribute to and exacerbate negative health behaviors that affect cognitive ability; and
3. Disability may reciprocally affect the determinants of cognitive deficits and depressive symptoms. See **Fig. 1** for a summary.

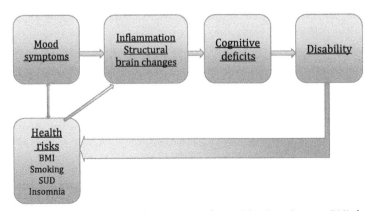

Fig. 1. Pathways between bipolar depression and cognitive impairment. BMI, body mass index; SUD, substance use disorder.

These pathways are speculative and not yet confirmed by longitudinal study; they are also not mutually exclusive yet produce unique implications for treatment. The evidence for these possibilities is reviewed in the following section.

Evidence for a Direct Pathway from Bipolar Depression to Cognitive Impairment

One direct neurobiological pathway from cumulative exposure to affective symptoms to cognition may be chronic stress-induced dysregulation of the immune system. Individuals with BD show an abnormal inflammatory profile, characterized by altered levels of both proinflammatory and antiinflammatory cytokines. Studies that have investigated the effects of mood state on inflammatory cytokines and have reported both upregulation and downregulation in these markers during depression, including C-reactive protein (CRP), interleukin 6 (IL-6), and tumor necrosis factor α (TNF-α).[29–32] There is some evidence to suggest that patterns of inflammation differ between mood states. Mania seems to produce more pronounced increase across many inflammatory markers compared with patients in depressed or euthymic phases of the disorder. Ortiz-Dominguez and colleagues[33] reported that depressed patients with BD in their sample showed increased IL-6 and TNF-α and decreased IL-2 levels. In contrast, mania was associated with increases in TNF-α and IL-4 and decreases in IL-1 and IL-2 levels. Thus, although BD seems to dysregulate inflammation across mood states, there is also some literature to suggest potential phasic differences in specific inflammatory cytokines.

Some preliminary investigations have highlighted the deleterious effect of a dysregulated inflammatory state on cognition. One study[34] reported negative correlations between CRP expression and immediate memory, language, and attention in BD. Another group[35] reported that worse performance on a task of delayed auditory verbal memory was associated with higher levels of TNF-α in a sample of patients with BD. Associations between cognition and inflammation have also been reported in psychiatrically healthy adults,[36,37] and levels of IL-6 predicted future cognitive decline, particularly in those with increased genetic risk for cognitive impairment. These largely cross-sectional studies indicate that alterations in specific inflammatory cytokines, particularly those shown to be dysregulated during the depressive phase of the disorder, may contribute to cognitive impairment in BD.

Neuroimaging findings have elucidated abnormal neural activity as well as altered white and gray matter organization in BD. Compromised white matter seems to be the most robust finding, and studies[38] have reported widespread alterations in white matter integrity. Importantly, these alterations are associated with deficits in processing speed, executive functioning, verbal fluency, and regulation of emotion.[39] A recent diffusion tensor imaging study[40] reported that alterations in white matter integrity were associated with poorer verbal fluency in a sample of depressed bipolar patients. Inflammation may contribute to white matter changes by inducing changes in myelin integrity and vascular permeability. Some studies have reported a negative relationship between proinflammatory cytokines and white matter integrity in healthy older adults[41] and patients with schizophrenia.[42] A review of the current evidence, although limited,[43] suggests that the prefrontal cortex, corpus callosum, and temporal lobe may be particularly vulnerable to inflammation in patients diagnosed with major depressive disorder.

There is some evidence to support the role of the number and severity of depressive episodes in development of white matter disease. Studies have shown associations between more symptoms of depression and greater white matter compromise in the anterior thalamic radiation and the corpus callosum.[44] Depressed individuals with BD also have greater compromise in the left cingulate subgyrus, the posterior limb of the right internal capsule, and the right parietal white matter tracts compared with euthymic patients with BD.[45] There is also some evidence to suggest a larger degree of white matter alteration in bipolar depression compared with unipolar depression, particularly in the corpus callosum,[46,47] indicating that individuals with BD may experience a similar, yet more severe, pathophysiologic disease course.

Evidence for an Indirect Pathway from Bipolar Depression to Health Risks to Cognitive Impairment

The alarmingly high prevalence of medical comorbidities in BD led many investigators to conclude that BD is a multisystem disease affecting a diverse array of organs beyond the brain. In addition to the direct impacts of the illness on immune function and other systems that influence brain function, indirect pathways that interact with mood symptoms include poor health behaviors, and other risk factors that may affect cognition. These factors include diet and physical activity, smoking and substance use, and potential iatrogenic effects of medication used to treat symptoms.

Obesity

Approximately 60% of people with BD are overweight (defined as a body mass index [BMI, calculated as weight in kilograms divided by the square of height in meters] >25 kg/m^2) and 20% to 40% obese (defined as a BMI >30 kg/m^{248}). These figures are high compared with those in the general US adult population (http://www.cdc.gov/nchs/fastats/obesity-overweight.htm). There are several risk factors for obesity, with patients with BD less likely to report recommended levels of physical activity and intake of fruits and vegetables. In addition, some of the medications used to treat BD are associated with weight gain and adiposity.

Data on the impact of obesity on cognition in BD are emerging, and studies have indicated the impact of obesity on both brain structural and functional changes as well as inflammatory markers. Depp and colleagues[49] examined the association of overweight and obesity with cognition in a sample of outpatients with BD and, adjusting for sociodemographic and clinical covariates, found a stepwise association with increasing evidence for impairment in overweight and obese patients. The difference in cognitive functioning between obese and normal weight patients was substantial (Cohen $d = 0.43$) and greater than observed in a comparison sample of obese, overweight, and normal weight patients with schizophrenia.

Work has begun to explore the link between diet, inflammation, and cognition in BD. Several studies have reported a higher prevalence of a Western diet (eg, red meat, refined carbohydrates, and processed foods) among depressed individuals,[50–53] including those diagnosed with BD.[54] Western diets have been linked to increased concentration of IL-6 and CRP inflammatory cytokines[50,55] and a reduction of glucose and metabolic transport in hippocampal regions in rats.[56] Conversely, middle-aged individuals adherent to a Mediterranean diet were associated with reduced levels of these same cytokines[57] and lower prevalence of metabolic syndrome[58] and cardiovascular disorders.[59] Thus, there is some preliminary evidence that suggests that dietary patterns may alter inflammatory profiles.

Physical Activity

Several epidemiologic studies indicate that people with BD are less likely than healthy comparators to engage in recommended levels of physical activity,[60] including those measured by objective ambulatory monitoring devices.[61,62] There is substantial evidence for an association between diminished physical activity and incidence of depressive symptoms, and reciprocal relationships have been observed in a longitudinal study of adolescents,[63] with increases in depression predicting later diminished physical activity. Self-reported physical activity studies[64] have indicated that less frequent exercise is associated with greater depression and lower quality of life, whereas increased activity predicts greater manic symptoms.

Substance Use

Rates of comorbid substance use in BD range from 20% to 60% across different samples.[65] Although the self-medication hypothesis of substance use in BD does not explain all of the comorbidity between affective and substance-related symptoms, there is research[66] to suggest that patients report use of substances to attempt to ameliorate depressive symptoms. Chronic substance use, particularly alcohol, has been shown to negatively affect several cognitive domains in BD, including executive functioning and memory.[67] Many of the deficits linked to chronic alcohol use have also been shown to be present in substance-free patients with BD, and some investigators suggest that comorbid substance use disorder and BD may have an additive effect on cognitive impairment. For example, one study[68,69] reported that euthymic patients with BD with a history of alcohol dependence show greater executive dysfunction compared with patients with BD without a history of use. Although several translational models have indicated the potential benefits of nicotine on brain function, there is mounting evidence that cigarette smoking is associated with cognitive deterioration. Depp and colleagues[70] examined the association of current smoking and lifetime smoking patterns with cognition in BD. Current smokers showed worse cognitive performance, and there was a modest negative association with between pack-years and global cognitive performance. Patients who had ceased smoking did not differ in cognitive performance from never smokers.

Sleep

As many as 70% of patients with BD have sleep problems even when euthymic. A study[71] found that 100% of patients experienced insomnia and 78% experienced hypersomnia during bipolar depression. Eidelman and colleagues[72] found that a greater number of past depressive episodes was associated with greater sleep disturbance. Conversely, euthymic patients culled from the large STEP-BD (Systematic Treatment Enhancement Program for Bipolar Disorder) trial[73] who had evidence of sleep disturbance were more at risk for mood episode recurrence. Few studies have examined the association between sleep and cognitive function in BD, although many studies have linked insomnia and worse cognition in other populations. Thus, strong connections between mood symptoms, sleep problems, and cognitive impairment in BD seem plausible. As with all of the risk factors described earlier, it is unclear if sleep mediates the associations between cognitive impairment, symptoms, and function or if aberrant sleep and cognitive impairments derive from the same neurobiological diathesis (eg, disrupted circadian rhythms).[74] Moreover, sleep problems also likely heavily exacerbate other health risk factors listed earlier; patients frequently use alcohol, prescription medications, and illicit substances to self-medicate sleep problems and subsequently further alter sleep architecture. Diminished physical activity may occur among patients with insomnia because of diminished energy, and poorer diet and obesity may be exacerbated through alterations to appetitive hormones associated with sleep problems.

Psychosocial Disabilities May Reciprocally Increase Depression and Cognitive Impairment

A less-discussed possibility in models of the predictors of disability in BD is that disability may reciprocally diminish cognitive function and increase depression. For example, although little studied in BD, engagement in cognitively stimulating activities has been studied extensively as a protective factor in cognitive functioning in healthy aging. Higher educational attainment and engagement in cognitively complex occupations seem to forestall cognitive decline, and greater engagement in cognitively sedentary activities such as watching television seems to be associated with increased risk of cognitive decline.[75] These findings have led to the concept of such behaviors as contributing to cognitive reserve and as protection against the age-associated deterioration in brain structure and function. It is evident that depressive symptoms predict diminished engagement in cognitively stimulating activities and vice versa,[76] and in patients with BD, participation in the workforce and potentially mentally challenging activity are both reduced.

In the general population, people with more robust and supportive social networks experience diminished risk of cognitive decline when followed prospectively.[77] These effects have been examined in studies that account for potential reciprocal effects of cognition on social functioning. Mechanisms of this association are unclear but may include that interpersonal relationships may provide cognitive challenges that enhance cognitive reserve and that strong social relations may buffer neurochemical effects of stress on cognitive deterioration. Numerous studies[78] have indicated that the social networks of people with BD are depleted compared with healthy control individuals, and social strain and negative interactions are increased.

Disability may influence depression and cognition in BD through the deleterious effects of poverty. BD is associated with higher rates of poverty and reliance on disability income, and socioeconomic factors may contribute substantially to the excess mortality experienced by people with BD by diminishing access to healthy diets, safe places for physical activity, and means of cognitive stimulation.

INTERVENTIONS TO REMEDIATE COGNITIVE IMPAIRMENT IN BIPOLAR DEPRESSION

The optimization of therapies for bipolar depression remains a critical challenge. Moreover, there have been few randomized controlled trials of any pharmacologic or nonpharmacologic therapies designed to enhance cognitive abilities in BD. Nonetheless, there are several potential intervention strategies that are relevant to discuss when considering the junction of cognitive impairment and depression, examining the broader literature outside BD and early-stage studies. In the following section, treatments are reviewed that have evidence for at least 1 of the following: (1) positive impact on both bipolar depression and cognitive ability, (2) mitigation of hypothesized biological mechanisms (eg, inflammation) that undergird depression and cognitive impairment, and (3) successful targeting of a risk factor associated with increased risk for cognitive impairment and more severe depression.

Pharmacologic Treatments

No agents for cognitive enhancement in BD have been approved by the US Food and Drug Administration (FDA). Given the emerging focus on inflammation in the pathophysiology of life-course models BD, an increasing number of antiinflammatory agents have been examined as potential adjunctive treatments for cognitive enhancement.[79] These agents include lithium and valproate, which suppress IL-6. A variety of other agents have been either evaluated or proposed as adjuvant therapies to diminish inflammation, including omega-3 fatty acids, aspirin, nonsteroidal antiinflammatory drugs, and N-acetylcysteine, as well as tetracyclic antibiotics (eg, minocycline), monoclonal antibodies (eg, TNF-α inhibitors), and phytochemicals (eg, cumin). A recent excellent review by Rosenblat and colleagues[79] described the mechanism and current status of trials of these agents in targeting unipolar and bipolar depression. Tempering enthusiasm is that several therapies have been evaluated as targets to prevent cognitive decline in normal aging, and despite strong observational associations (eg, omega-3 fatty acids), randomized trials have proved disappointing.[80] Nonetheless, in contrast to normal aging, patients with BD are a substantially more enriched sample in which to show the impact of antiinflammatory agents for both bipolar depression and cognitive function, for the reasons detailed earlier.

Other agents that have been used to target cognition may also have antidepressant effects and vice versa. For example, Burdick and colleagues[81] reported results of a trial of pramipexole targeting cognitive functioning in bipolar I and found in post hoc analyses a benefit among patients with cognitive impairment at baseline. Pramipexole has also been examined as a treatment of bipolar depression. Trials typically attempt to isolate the impact of agents on cognitive enhancement by restriction to euthymic patients or examining whether (subsyndromal) depressive symptoms moderated or mediated the impact of the agent. However, it may be possible to consider agents with broad-spectrum impact on both cognitive impairment and bipolar depression.

Cognitive Training and Remediation

Two recent randomized trials[82,83] suggested limited impact of broadly targeted cognitive remediation on objective cognitive performance in euthymic patients with BD, despite earlier open trials indicating some enhancement of cognitive ability. Nonetheless, in the larger trial reported by Torrent and colleagues[82] involving an intervention that provided psychoeducation and behavioral practice of cognitive compensatory techniques, psychosocial functioning was enhanced to a significant degree compared with a symptom-focused psychoeducation group.

More targeted cognitive training, not yet tested in BD, has shown some ability to enhance both cognitive function and depressive symptoms. In the large ACTIVE (Advanced Cognitive Training for Independent and Vital Elderly) study, a clinical trial of several cognitive training interventions evaluated in older adults, speed-of-processing training was associated with a 30% reduction in the likelihood of clinically significant increases in depressive symptoms over 5 years of follow-up.[84] Emerging arenas at the boundary of cognitive training include cognitive bias modification, social cognitive skills training, and interventions focused on regulation of emotion. These areas typically target aberrant or extreme preconscious cognitive phenomena (eg, overgeneral memory biases in depression) and have been associated with typically short-term improvements in biases and some impact on depressive symptoms. Given the emerging understanding of the neural basis of emotion in BD, these interventions hold promise as potential adjunctive treatments.[85]

Physical Activity and Weight Loss Interventions

Comprehensive weight loss interventions targeting energy balance and dietary intake have been effective in reducing weight in samples of people with serious mental illness.[86] Physical activity is frequently mentioned as a generally low-risk broad-spectrum intervention that could affect inflammatory processes, metabolism, depressive symptoms, and cognitive function. Several reviews[87] have described the status of the literature on physical activity interventions in BD, and most have concluded promise but need for more well-designed trials. There are trials[88] that have indicated positive impact of physical activity interventions on cognition in patients with depression and schizophrenia.

Treatment of Insomnia

Recent preliminary work has shown impressive effects of adapted cognitive behavioral therapy (CBT) for Insomnia (CBT-I) in BD. Lee and Harvey[89] reported pilot data from an open trial of an 8-session intervention targeting insomnia in BD, and in addition to improving sleep function at 6 months, reduced rates of mood relapse and diminished functional impairment were observed. It would be important to determine if such an approach might also reduce cognitive impairment.

Compensating for Cognitive Impairment in Learning-Based Therapies

Cognitive impairments likely limit the degree to which patients retain information and subsequently benefit from learning-based psychotherapies like CBT that target depressive symptoms. In the study by Lee and Harvey[89] regarding CBT-I described earlier, an interesting subanalysis showed that patients with insomnia recalled less than 20% of CBT material. Mobile devices may provide a novel means of augmenting psychotherapies to enhance recall and community engagement in therapeutically relevant activities. Depp and colleagues[90] evaluated a mobile augmented intervention called PRISM (Personalized Real-Time Intervention for Stabilizing Mood), which involved brief psychoeducation combined with automated frequent assessments and linked personalized reminders to engage in coping strategies identified during in-person training. Compared with a condition in which patients only participated in face-to-face training and completed paper-and-pencil mood charts, patients who received PRISM experienced a significantly greater reduction in bipolar depression at poststudy.

SUMMARY

There is both remarkable challenge and opportunity at the intersection of bipolar depression and cognitive impairment. A pessimistic viewpoint would emphasize that, despite contributing to most of the personal and economic burden of BD, providers have few treatment options to offer their patients. Remarkably, only 3 agents are approved by the FDA for acute bipolar depression and no agents are FDA approved for cognitive enhancement.

An optimistic view would be that research has now identified shared determinants and treatment avenues for biological mechanisms that undergird bipolar depression and cognition, such as chronic inflammation. Work in this area has opened a host of novel pharmacologic and nonpharmacologic treatment possibilities that may simultaneously target these two pernicious aspects of the illness and point to preventive approaches to forestall cognitive decline. Available to clinicians are efficacious interventions that reduce health risks associated with both depression and cognitive impairment, such as physical activity, cognitive behavioral treatment of insomnia, and weight loss intervention. Novel psychotherapeutic treatments may circumvent or compensate for cognitive deficits through technology and could provide more substantial impact on bipolar depression. These opportunities make BD a model condition in which to enhance understanding and develop treatments for co-occurring cognitive impairment and depression.

REFERENCES

1. Burdick KE, Goldberg TE, Cornblatt BA, et al. The MATRICS consensus cognitive battery in patients with bipolar I disorder. Neuropsychopharmacology 2011;36(8): 1587–92.

2. Simonsen C, Sundet K, Vaskinn A, et al. Neurocognitive profiles in bipolar I and bipolar II disorder: differences in pattern and magnitude of dysfunction. Bipolar Disord 2008;10(2):245–55.
3. Dittmann S, Hennig-Fast K, Gerber S, et al. Cognitive functioning in euthymic bipolar I and bipolar II patients. Bipolar Disord 2008;10(8):877–87.
4. Martinez-Aran A, Torrent C, Tabares-Seisdedos R, et al. Neurocognitive impairment in bipolar patients with and without history of psychosis. J Clin Psychiatry 2008;69(2):233–9.
5. Torres IJ, Boudreau VG, Yatham LN. Neuropsychological functioning in euthymic bipolar disorder: a meta-analysis. Acta Psychiatr Scand Suppl 2007;434:17–26.
6. Arts B, Jabben N, Krabbendam L, et al. Meta-analyses of cognitive functioning in euthymic bipolar patients and their first-degree relatives. Psychol Med 2008; 38(06):771–85.
7. Burdick K, Russo M, Frangou S, et al. Empirical evidence for discrete neurocognitive subgroups in bipolar disorder: clinical implications. Psychol Med 2014; 44(14):3083–96.
8. Samamé C, Martino DJ, Strejilevich SA. An individual task meta-analysis of social cognition in euthymic bipolar disorders. J Affect Disord 2015;173(0):146–53.
9. Krabbendam L, Arts BM, Van Os J, et al. Cognitive functioning in patients with schizophrenia and bipolar disorder: a quantitative review. Schizophr Res 2005; 80(2–3):137–49.
10. Taylor Tavares JV, Clark L, Cannon DM, et al. Distinct profiles of neurocognitive function in unmedicated unipolar depression and bipolar II depression. Biol Psychiatry 2007;62(8):917–24.
11. Xu G, Lin K, Rao D, et al. Neuropsychological performance in bipolar I, bipolar II and unipolar depression patients: a longitudinal, naturalistic study. J Affect Disord 2012;136(3):328–39.
12. Cerullo MA, Eliassen JC, Smith CT, et al. Bipolar I disorder and major depressive disorder show similar brain activation during depression. Bipolar Disord 2014; 16(7):703–12.
13. Kurtz MM, Gerraty RT. A meta-analytic investigation of neurocognitive deficits in bipolar illness: profile and effects of clinical state. Neuropsychology 2009;23(5): 551.
14. Martinez-Aran A, Vieta E, Reinares M, et al. Cognitive function across manic or hypomanic, depressed, and euthymic states in bipolar disorder. Am J Psychiatry 2004;161:262–70.
15. Van Rheenen TE, Rossell SL. An empirical evaluation of the MATRICS consensus cognitive battery in bipolar disorder. Bipolar Disord 2014;16(3):318–25.
16. Malhi GS, Ivanovski B, Hadzi-Pavlovic D, et al. Neuropsychological deficits and functional impairment in bipolar depression, hypomania and euthymia. Bipolar Disord 2007;9(1–2):114–25.
17. Muralidharan K, Torres IJ, Silveira LE, et al. Impact of depressive episodes on cognitive deficits in early bipolar disorder: data from the Systematic Treatment Optimization Programme for Early Mania (STOP-EM). Br J Psychiatry 2014; 205(1):36–43.
18. Goodwin GM, Martinez-Aran A, Glahn DC, et al. Cognitive impairment in bipolar disorder: neurodevelopment or neurodegeneration? An ECNP expert meeting report. Eur Neuropsychopharmacol 2008;18(11):787–93.
19. Berk M, Kapczinski F, Andreazza AC, et al. Pathways underlying neuroprogression in bipolar disorder: focus on inflammation, oxidative stress and neurotrophic factors. Neurosci Biobehav Rev 2011;35(3):804–17.

20. Robinson LJ, Ferrier IN. Evolution of cognitive impairment in bipolar disorder: a systematic review of cross-sectional evidence. Bipolar Disord 2006;8(2):103–16.

21. Zahodne LB, Stern Y, Manly JJ. Depressive symptoms precede memory decline, but not vice versa, in non-demented older adults. J Am Geriatr Soc 2014;62(1): 130–4.

22. Berk M, Berk L, Dodd S, et al. Stage managing bipolar disorder. Bipolar Disord 2014;16(5):471–7.

23. Depp CA, Mausbach BT, Harmell AL, et al. Meta-analysis of the association between cognitive abilities and everyday functioning in bipolar disorder. Bipolar Disord 2012;14(3):217–26.

24. Judd LL, Akiskal HS, Schettler PJ, et al. Psychosocial disability in the course of bipolar I and II disorders: a prospective, comparative, longitudinal study. Arch Gen Psychiatry 2005;62(12):1322–30.

25. Bowie CR, Depp C, McGrath JA, et al. Prediction of real-world functional disability in chronic mental disorders: a comparison of schizophrenia and bipolar disorder. Am J Psychiatry 2010;167(9):1116–24.

26. Bonnín CM, Martínez-Arán A, Torrent C, et al. Clinical and neurocognitive predictors of functional outcome in bipolar euthymic patients: a long-term, follow-up study. J Affect Disord 2010;121(1–2):156–60.

27. Depp CA, Mausbach BT, Bowie C, et al. Determinants of occupational and residential functioning in bipolar disorder. J Affect Disord 2012;136(3):812–8.

28. Harvey PD, Paschall G, Depp C. Factors influencing self-assessment of cognition and functioning in bipolar disorder: a preliminary study. Cogn Neuropsychiatry 2015;20(4):361–71.

29. Brietzke E, Stertz L, Fernandes BS, et al. Comparison of cytokine levels in depressed, manic and euthymic patients with bipolar disorder. J Affect Disord 2009;116(3):214–7.

30. De Berardis D, Conti CM, Campanella D, et al. Evaluation of C-reactive protein and total serum cholesterol in adult patients with bipolar disorder. Int J Immunopathol Pharmacol 2008;21(2):319–24.

31. Kapczinski F, Dal-Pizzol F, Teixeira AL, et al. Peripheral biomarkers and illness activity in bipolar disorder. J Psychiatr Res 2011;45(2):156–61.

32. O'Brien SM, Scully P, Scott LV, et al. Cytokine profiles in bipolar affective disorder: focus on acutely ill patients. J Affect Disord 2006;90(2–3):263–7.

33. Ortiz-Dominguez A, Hernandez ME, Berlanga C, et al. Immune variations in bipolar disorder: phasic differences. Bipolar Disord 2007;9(6):596–602.

34. Dickerson F, Stallings C, Origoni A, et al. Elevated C-reactive protein and cognitive deficits in individuals with bipolar disorder. J Affect Disord 2013;150(2): 456–9.

35. Doganavsargil-Baysal O, Cinemre B, Aksoy UM, et al. Levels of TNF-alpha, soluble TNF receptors (sTNFR1, sTNFR2), and cognition in bipolar disorder. Hum Psychopharmacol 2013;28(2):160–7.

36. Teunissen CE, van Boxtel MP, Bosma H, et al. Inflammation markers in relation to cognition in a healthy aging population. J Neuroimmunol 2003;134(1–2): 142–50.

37. Wright CB, Sacco RL, Rundek T, et al. Interleukin-6 is associated with cognitive function: the Northern Manhattan Study. J Stroke Cerebrovasc Dis 2006;15(1): 34–8.

38. Nortje G, Stein DJ, Radua J, et al. Systematic review and voxel-based meta-analysis of diffusion tensor imaging studies in bipolar disorder. J Affect Disord 2013;150(2): 192–200.

39. Bearden CE, Hoffman KM, Cannon TD. The neuropsychology and neuroanatomy of bipolar affective disorder: a critical review. Bipolar Disord 2001;3(3):106–50 [discussion: 151–3].
40. Bauer IE, Ouyang A, Mwangi B, et al. Reduced white matter integrity and verbal fluency impairment in young adults with bipolar disorder: a diffusion tensor imaging study. J Psychiatr Res 2015;62:115–22.
41. Bettcher BM, Watson CL, Walsh CM, et al. Interleukin-6, age, and corpus callosum integrity. PLoS One 2014;9(9):e106521.
42. Prasad KM, Upton CH, Nimgaonkar VL, et al. Differential susceptibility of white matter tracts to inflammatory mediators in schizophrenia: an integrated DTI study. Schizophr Res 2015;161(1):119–25.
43. Frodl T, Amico F. Is there an association between peripheral immune markers and structural/functional neuroimaging findings? Prog Neuropsychopharmacol Biol Psychiatry 2014;48:295–303.
44. Sussmann JE, Lymer GKS, McKirdy J, et al. White matter abnormalities in bipolar disorder and schizophrenia detected using diffusion tensor magnetic resonance imaging. Bipolar Disord 2009;11(1):11–8.
45. Zanetti M, Jackowski M, Versace A, et al. State-dependent microstructural white matter changes in bipolar I depression. Eur Arch Psychiatry Clin Neurosci 2009; 259(6):316–28.
46. Wise T, Radua J, Nortje G, et al. Voxel-based meta-analytical evidence of structural disconnectivity in major depression and bipolar disorder. Biol Psychiatry 2015. [Epub ahead of print].
47. Yamada S, Takahashi S, Ukai S, et al. Microstructural abnormalities in anterior callosal fibers and their relationship with cognitive function in major depressive disorder and bipolar disorder: a tract-specific analysis study. J Affect Disord 2015;174:542–8.
48. McElroy SL, Keck PE. Obesity in bipolar disorder: an overview. Curr Psychiatry Rep 2012;14(6):1–9.
49. Depp CA, Strassnig M, Mausbach BT, et al. Association of obesity and treated hypertension and diabetes with cognitive ability in bipolar disorder and schizophrenia. Bipolar Disord 2014;16(4):422–31.
50. Berk M, Williams LJ, Jacka FN, et al. So depression is an inflammatory disease, but where does the inflammation come from? BMC Med 2013;11:200.
51. Jacka FN, Pasco JA, Mykletun A, et al. Association of Western and traditional diets with depression and anxiety in women. Am J Psychiatry 2010;167(3):305–11.
52. Jacka FN, Mykletun A, Berk M, et al. The association between habitual diet quality and the common mental disorders in community-dwelling adults: the Hordaland Health Study. Psychosom Med 2011;73(6):483–90.
53. Nanri A, Kimura Y, Matsushita Y, et al. Dietary patterns and depressive symptoms among Japanese men and women. Eur J Clin Nutr 2010;64(8):832–9.
54. Jacka FN, Pasco JA, Mykletun A, et al. Diet quality in bipolar disorder in a population-based sample of women. J Affect Disord 2011;129(1–3):332–7.
55. Lopez-Garcia E, Schulze MB, Fung TT, et al. Major dietary patterns are related to plasma concentrations of markers of inflammation and endothelial dysfunction. Am J Clin Nutr 2004;80(4):1029–35.
56. Hargrave SL, Davidson TL, Lee TJ, et al. Brain and behavioral perturbations in rats following Western diet access. Appetite 2015;93:35–43.
57. Dai J, Miller AH, Bremner JD, et al. Adherence to the Mediterranean diet is inversely associated with circulating interleukin-6 among middle-aged men: a twin study. Circulation 2008;117(2):169–75.

58. Viscogliosi G, Cipriani E, Liguori ML, et al. Mediterranean dietary pattern adherence: associations with prediabetes, metabolic syndrome, and related microinflammation. Metab Syndr Relat Disord 2013;11(3):210–6.
59. Ginter E, Simko V. Recent data on Mediterranean diet, cardiovascular disease, cancer, diabetes and life expectancy. Bratisl Lek Listy 2015;116(6):346–8.
60. Vancampfort D, Correll CU, Probst M, et al. A review of physical activity correlates in patients with bipolar disorder. J Affect Disord 2013;145(3):285–91.
61. Krane-Gartiser K, Henriksen TE, Morken G, et al. Actigraphic assessment of motor activity in acutely admitted inpatients with bipolar disorder. PLoS One 2014; 9(2):e89574.
62. Janney CA, Fagiolini A, Swartz HA, et al. Are adults with bipolar disorder active? Objectively measured physical activity and sedentary behavior using accelerometry. J Affect Disord 2014;152-154:498–504.
63. Jerstad SJ, Boutelle KN, Ness KK, et al. Prospective reciprocal relations between physical activity and depression in female adolescents. J Consult Clin Psychol 2010;78(2):268.
64. Sylvia LG, Friedman ES, Kocsis JH, et al. Association of exercise with quality of life and mood symptoms in a comparative effectiveness study of bipolar disorder. J Affect Disord 2013;151(2):722–7.
65. Nesvag R, Knudsen GP, Bakken IJ, et al. Substance use disorders in schizophrenia, bipolar disorder, and depressive illness: a registry-based study. Soc Psychiatry Psychiatr Epidemiol 2015;50(8):1267–76.
66. Bizzarri JV, Sbrana A, Rucci P, et al. The spectrum of substance abuse in bipolar disorder: reasons for use, sensation seeking and substance sensitivity. Bipolar Disord 2007;9(3):213–20.
67. Balanza-Martinez V, Crespo-Facorro B, Gonzalez-Pinto A, et al. Bipolar disorder comorbid with alcohol use disorder: focus on neurocognitive correlates. Front Physiol 2015;6:108.
68. Levy B, Weiss RD. Neurocognitive impairment and psychosis in bipolar disorder during early remission from an acute episode of mood disturbance. J Clin Psychiatry 2010;71(2):201–6.
69. Levy B, Weiss RD. Cognitive functioning in bipolar and co-occurring substance use disorders: a missing piece in the puzzle. Harv Rev Psychiatry 2009;17(3):226–30.
70. Depp CA, Bowie CR, Mausbach BT, et al. Current smoking is associated with worse cognitive and adaptive functioning in serious mental illness. Acta Psychiatr Scand 2015;131(5):333–41.
71. Harvey AG, Talbot LS, Gershon A. Sleep disturbance in bipolar disorder across the lifespan. Clin Psychol 2009;16(2):256–77.
72. Eidelman P, Talbot LS, Gruber J, et al. Sleep, illness course, and concurrent symptoms in inter-episode bipolar disorder. J Behav Ther Exp Psychiatry 2010; 41(2):145–9.
73. Gruber J, Harvey AG, Wang PW, et al. Sleep functioning in relation to mood, function, and quality of life at entry to the Systematic Treatment Enhancement Program for Bipolar Disorder (STEP-BD). J Affect Disord 2009;114(1–3):41–9.
74. Boland EM, Alloy LB. Sleep disturbance and cognitive deficits in bipolar disorder: toward an integrated examination of disorder maintenance and functional impairment. Clin Psychol Rev 2013;33(1):33–44.
75. Stern Y. Cognitive reserve in ageing and Alzheimer's disease. Lancet Neurol 2012;11(11):1006–12.
76. Zhai L, Zhang Y, Zhang D. Sedentary behaviour and the risk of depression: a meta-analysis. Br J Sports Med 2015;49(11):705–9.

77. James BD, Wilson RS, Barnes LL, et al. Late-life social activity and cognitive decline in old age. J Int Neuropsychol Soc 2011;17(06):998–1005.
78. Eidelman P, Gershon A, Kaplan K, et al. Social support and social strain in inter-episode bipolar disorder. Bipolar Disord 2012;14(6):628–40.
79. Rosenblat JD, Cha DS, Mansur RB, et al. Inflamed moods: a review of the interactions between inflammation and mood disorders. Prog Neuropsychopharmacol Biol Psychiatry 2014;53(0):23–34.
80. Cederholm T, Salem N, Palmblad J. ω-3 Fatty acids in the prevention of cognitive decline in humans. Adv Nutr 2013;4(6):672–6.
81. Burdick KE, Braga RJ, Nnadi CU, et al. Placebo-controlled adjunctive trial of pramipexole in patients with bipolar disorder: targeting cognitive dysfunction. J Clin Psychiatry 2012;73(1):103–12.
82. Torrent C, Bonnin Cdel M, Martínez-Arán A, et al. Efficacy of functional remediation in bipolar disorder: a multicenter randomized controlled study. Am J Psychiatry 2013;170(8):852–9.
83. Demant KM, Vinberg M, Kessing LV, et al. Effects of short-term cognitive remediation on cognitive dysfunction in partially or fully remitted individuals with bipolar disorder: results of a randomised controlled trial. PLoS One 2015;10(6):e0127955.
84. Wolinsky FD, Vander Weg MW, Martin R, et al. The effect of speed-of-processing training on depressive symptoms in ACTIVE. J Gerontol A Biol Sci Med Sci 2009; 64(4):468–72.
85. Joormann J, Quinn ME. Cognitive processes and emotion regulation in depression. Depress Anxiety 2014;31(4):308–15.
86. Daumit GL, Dickerson FB, Wang N-Y, et al. A behavioral weight-loss intervention in persons with serious mental illness. N Engl J Med 2013;368(17):1594–602.
87. Malchow B, Reich-Erkelenz D, Oertel-Knöchel V, et al. The effects of physical exercise in schizophrenia and affective disorders. Eur Arch Psychiatry Clin Neurosci 2013;263(6):451–67.
88. Kucyi A, Alsuwaidan MT, Liauw SS, et al. Aerobic physical exercise as a possible treatment for neurocognitive dysfunction in bipolar disorder. Postgrad Med 2010; 122(6):107–16.
89. Lee JY, Harvey AG. Memory for therapy in bipolar disorder and comorbid insomnia. J Consult Clin Psychol 2015;83(1):92.
90. Depp CA, Ceglowski J, Wang VC, et al. Augmenting psychoeducation with a mobile intervention for bipolar disorder: a randomized controlled trial. J Affect Disord 2015;174(0):23–30.

Suicide Behaviors in Bipolar Disorder

A Review and Update for the Clinician

John L. Beyer, MD*, Richard H. Weisler, MD

KEYWORDS

- Bipolar • Depression • Suicide • Lithium • Antidepressants • Risk factors

KEY POINTS

- Bipolar disorder is highly associated with suicide behaviors; among all the psychiatric illnesses, bipolar disorder seems to have the highest risk for suicide attempts and completions.
- The greatest risk factors for suicide completion are previous suicide attempts and a family history of suicide.
- Although frequently used to treat bipolar depression, antidepressants may have a suicide-provoking effect in younger adults and adolescents.
- Lithium seems to have suicide-preventing effects.

INTRODUCTION

Suicide is a major public health issue. In 2012, an estimated 804,000 people worldwide committed suicide,[1] accounting for 1.5% of all deaths and making it the 15th leading cause of death. However, owing to the significant stigma associated with suicide, various countries' laws about suicide, and even basic reporting/classification issues, it is believed that the actual number of deaths by suicide is much higher. Further, for every completed suicide, there are many more who attempt suicide, often straining resources and social network fabrics.

In 2013 in the United States, there were 41,149 suicides, an average of 113 each day. This makes suicide the 10th leading cause of death overall, although it is the second leading cause of death in persons age 15 to 34 (just behind unintentional injuries), and the third leading cause of death in persons age 10 to 14.[2] General population surveys of the United States document a suicide attempt rate of 0.6%, and a suicide ideation rate of 3.3%.[3]

Duke University Medical Center, Box 3519, Durham, NC 27710, USA
* Corresponding author. Duke University Medical Center, Box 3519, Durham, NC 27710.
E-mail address: john.beyer@dm.duke.edu

Psychiatr Clin N Am 39 (2016) 111–123
http://dx.doi.org/10.1016/j.psc.2015.09.002
0193-953X/16/$ – see front matter © 2016 Elsevier Inc. All rights reserved.

Suicide is a major concern to all clinicians treating psychiatric patients because it is a common endpoint for many patients with severe psychiatric illnesses. More than 90% of suicides occur in persons who have a Diagnostic & Statistical Manual–defined psychiatric illness.[4] The most commonly associated of these are the mood disorders—major depressive disorders and bipolar disorders—accounting for more than 60% of associated suicides. Many studies have suggested that the psychiatric illness with the highest prevalence of suicide behaviors is bipolar disorder.

This review provides the clinician an update on suicide behaviors in bipolar disorder treatment. We have attempted to identify the most commonly asked questions about suicide behavior, and review the current understanding available in this growing literature.

SUICIDE BEHAVIORS IN BIPOLAR DISORDER
When Researchers Discuss "Suicide Behaviors," to What Are They Referring?

One of the major difficulties in understanding the problem of suicide in our culture and in research studies is that suicide behaviors may be defined differently. For example, "Is every self-injurious act a suicide attempt?" or "At what point does preparation for suicide become an attempt?" Over the past 2 decades, researchers have adopted a more consistent language about suicide behaviors.[5] These include the following definitions.

Suicidal act
A self-injurious act committed by an individual with either explicit or implicit intent to die. If the outcome of a suicidal act is death, then it is called a completed suicide; otherwise, it is referred to as a suicide attempt.

Suicidal ideation
Suicidal ideation include thoughts about the desire, intent, and method for committing suicide. In this definition, the intensity of suicidal thoughts does not matter. They may range from the occasional fleeting thought to fulminate rumination and/or planning.

Suicide attempt
A self-injurious act committed with at least some intention to die. The amount of intention may vary, but by definition, as long as there is any intent to die associated with the act, it would be considered as an attempt.

Interrupted attempt
When the attempter is interrupted and prevented by outside circumstances from beginning self-injurious behaviors.

Aborted attempt
When the individual begins the suicidal act but stops before any destructive behavior has been completed.

It should be noted that even though the greatest predictor of suicide completion is previous suicide attempts,[6,7] there are significant differences globally between the much larger group of those who attempt suicide and the smaller number who complete suicide. Therefore, research data often differentiate the 2 groups as related but separate. In our review, we focus on the larger literature of suicide behaviors (ie, suicide ideation, attempt, completion), but we also identify specific differences among the behaviors.

What Is the Prevalence of Suicide Behaviors in Bipolar Disorder?

Several studies have attempted to assess the risk of suicide completion in patients with bipolar disorder. A systematic review of 34 studies found that the risk of suicide among bipolar subjects was 20 to 30 times greater than that for the general population,[8] although the rates differed based on individual bipolar sample populations. The rate of death by suicide for bipolar patients has been estimated to be 0.4% per year,[9] although extrapolation to a lifetime risk is uncertain.[10] Nordentoft and colleagues[11] looked at the risk of suicide after first psychiatric contact among a large Danish registry (>175,000 individuals) with a variety of mental illnesses over a 36-year period (median follow-up of 18 years). They found the absolute risk of suicide among patients with a diagnosis of bipolar disorder at first hospitalization is around 8% for men and 5% for women, which was the highest risk of suicide among all mental illnesses. The finding that bipolar disorder has the strongest association with suicide among various psychiatric conditions has been a repeated finding in the literature.[12,13] Some studies have even suggested that bipolar II disorder has an even higher association with suicide compared with bipolar I disorder, although more recent metaanalyses have not found this consistently.[10] Overall, suicide in bipolar disorder may account for up to one-quarter of all completed suicides.[12]

Rates of suicide attempts are also increased in bipolar disorder. The estimated annual risk of a suicide attempt was 0.9% per year. The lifetime risk for a suicide attempt in patients with bipolar disorder has been estimated at 25% to 50%.[14–17] Some researchers have expressed concern about the high lethality of suicide acts in bipolar disorder because of the much lower ratio of attempted suicide to completed suicide (approximately 3:1) compared with the general population (approximately 30:1).[18,19]

Why Do Patients with Bipolar Disorder Attempt or Commit Suicide?

The causes of suicide behaviors are complex and multiple. Suicide stands as the anchor point on a continuum from risk-taking behaviors, through various degrees and types of suicidal thinking, and ends with suicide attempts or completion.[20] However, the relationship between the stressful events of life, psychiatric illness, and suicide are not always straightforward. This can be observed by the fact that even extreme stressful life events by themselves do not necessarily lead to suicidal behaviors. Therefore, any model to explain suicide must account for the proximal factors (what is happening currently in a person's life) and distal factors (what has happened before) and their interaction.[21] Such observations have led to the stress–diathesis model of suicide behavior proposed by Mann and colleagues.[22] This model recognizes that the development of suicidal behavior involves a vulnerability (or diathesis) as distal risk factors that predispose individuals to suicidal behavior when under stress (proximal risk factors; **Fig. 1**). This model thus allows for the integration between underlying biological predispositions to suicide and the precipitants that may trigger it. Stress events could include the acute psychiatric illness, interpersonal problems, acute life events, and so on; whereas the distal factors may influence the predisposition to commit suicide, such as genetic vulnerability, compromised serotonergic functioning, temperamental variables (aggressiveness, impulsivity, hopelessness), substance abuse, chronic medical conditions, or even certain social factors (early death of a parent, social isolation, childhood abuse). The model postulates that suicide behavior is the result of the interaction between an individual's threshold for suicidal acts and the stressors that can lead to those behaviors.

RISK FACTORS FOR SUICIDE BEHAVIORS AND BIPOLAR DISORDER
What Then Are the Major Risk Factors in Suicide Behaviors?

As noted, suicide behavior is caused by or related to multiple factors that may have different importance from individual to individual. There are some general factors,

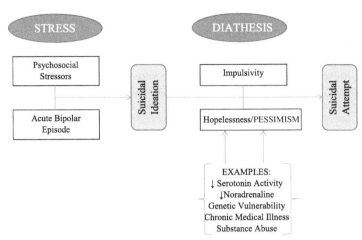

Fig. 1. Stress-diathesis model of suicide in bipolar disorder. ↓, decreased. (*Adapted from* Mann JJ, Waternaux C, Haas GL, et al. Toward a clinical model of suicidal behavior in psychiatric patients. Am J Psychiatry 1999;156:185.)

however, that may be more common and have a general higher risk than others. There are also some bipolar disease–specific factors that also contribute to increased suicide risk.

SOCIODEMOGRAPHIC FACTORS
Family History of Completed Suicide

In a recent metaanalysis evaluating correlates of suicide behavior in bipolar disorder, Schaffer and colleagues[10] found that the presence of first-degree family history of suicide had the strongest association with suicide deaths and attempts in bipolar disorder patients. This finding has been replicated repeatedly.[8,23] This finding supports the importance of both genetic and epigenetic factors and how they are integrated.[24] For example, Miklowitz and Chang[25] have found an association between family functioning and suicidality in youths with bipolar disorder, suggesting that bipolar disorder may involve a dysregulation of both mood and interpersonal processes where threats of harm occur both impulsively and/or instrumentally. Alternatively, suicide may be related to a shared environment that includes multiple risk factors, such as low quality of life.

Quality of Life/Stressful Life Events

Quality of life has long been known to be associated with suicidal behaviors in both the general population and in psychiatrically ill individuals. However, patients with bipolar disorder frequently show markedly impaired quality of life, even when clinically euthymic.[26,27] De Abreu and colleagues[26] have suggested that low quality of life may reflect poor coping skills and inadequate social support, which in turn increases the risk of suicide behaviors, although identifying and quantifying what is meant by "quality of life" needs further investigation.

Gender

In their metaanalysis of suicide correlates in bipolar disorder, Schaffer and colleagues[10] confirmed previous observations that female gender was associated with suicide attempts whereas male gender was associated with suicide completion.

This finding is consistent with gender differences found in all suicide behaviors and is not specific for bipolar disorder. However, the strength of the association may be less intense in bipolar disorder compared with the general population. Overall in bipolar disorder, men are twice as likely to die by suicide as compared with women compared with the general population, in which men are 4 times as likely to die by suicide compared with women. The corollary to this observation is that there is probably a higher suicide completion rate in women with bipolar disorder.

Age of Onset

Early onset illness has consistently been shown to be associated with a more severe course of illness in bipolar disorder.[28] Similarly, early age of onset is also associated with a higher likelihood of suicide attempts.[10] It is thought that this may represent either an increased genetic risk, more intense symptoms, or prolonged exposure to depressive episodes.[29] It should be noted that bipolar disorder has an earlier mean age of onset compared with unipolar depression.

Comorbidity

Studies have found consistently that there is a strong association between suicidal behaviors and psychiatric comorbidities. Comorbid anxiety disorders, substance use disorders, and Cluster B/borderline personality disorder are all associated with increased suicidal attempts.[10,30] This finding is especially concerning because almost two-thirds of all patients with bipolar disorder also struggle with either an anxiety disorder or substance abuse disorder or both. The exact causality is unclear. Some researchers suggest comorbid conditions reflect a more severe form of bipolar disorder. Others have suggested that, for the anxious bipolar patient, suicide thoughts may be a focus of increased ruminations[16,31] or a comorbid cluster B personality structure[32]; in contrast, the association with alcohol and drug use may be more mediated by increased impulsivity[33,34] or as markers of poor coping skills and inadequate social support.[26] Interestingly, 1 comorbid condition not associated with either a greater number of suicide attempts or completions is a history of psychosis.[10]

Hopelessness

An increasing amount of work has been done on psychological aspects of suicidal ideation, attempts, and completions. Recent reviews and metaanalyses have identified hopelessness as an important independent risk factor for suicide behavior.[35,36] Although the research construct of hopelessness is multifaceted, the gist of hopelessness among bipolar patients as a lack of positive future thinking is very important, possibly more important than the presence of negative future thinking.

Altitude

Regional variation in suicide behaviors has long been known to exist. Certain locations, especially in high-stress areas, have higher levels of suicide. Interestingly, researchers have noted that for the past 3 decades that suicide rates in the Intermountain West area of the United States has a higher suicide rate compared with lower altitude states.[37] This observation has been replicated by other researchers,[38,39] noting that altitude is an independent risk factor for suicide, even when controlling for gun ownership, rurality, age, and access to mental health providers. It has been hypothesized that changes in dopamine and serotonin may occur in the presence of hypoxia, possibly from the direct effect of altitude or because of underlying mitochondrial dysfunction that may be related to bipolar disorders.

BIPOLAR-SPECIFIC RISK FACTORS
Depression

In a metaanalysis of suicidal behavior correlates in bipolar patients, depressive polarity of the current or most recent mood episode had the strongest association with a suicide attempt.[10] Although it would come as no surprise that suicide attempts and completions occur primarily in the depressed state, this finding is striking in our attempt to understand suicide behaviors. Whatever reasons people may consider self-harm, the depressive state is one of the leading risk factors. Suicides during mania are relatively rare. However, several researchers have found that a broadly defined mixed state may actually be associated with the highest risk of suicide attempts per time period spent in a specific phase of illness,[40,41] as if negative self-thoughts, hopelessness, excessive guilt, and increased agitation/energy combine to create the highest risk of self-harm. It is possible that bipolar disorder may carry the highest association of suicidal behavior among psychiatric diseases for just those reasons.

Severity of Illness

One of the most challenging findings in bipolar disorder is the extent to which patients demonstrate active symptoms. For example, Judd and colleagues[42] in their study of mood charting over a grater than 12-year period found that bipolar I disorder patients spent an average of 46% of their days in a depressed mood/phase. Bipolar II patients had even a higher incidence of days spent in a depressed mood/phase.[43] Therefore, if being in a depressed phase of illness is a strong risk for suicide behavior, bipolar patients spend much of their time in a high-risk condition. Holma and colleagues[40] have suggested that the observed higher cumulative incidence of suicide attempts among patients with bipolar disorder than among those with a major depressive disorder was mostly owing to patients with bipolar disorder spending more time in high-risk illness phases, rather than to difference during these phases or to the bipolarity itself. Their suggestion is that diminishing the time spent in high-risk phases is crucial for prevention.

Polarity of First Episode

Interestingly, bipolar patients who had a depressive polarity of first mood episode were nearly twice as likely to attempt suicide. This has been a consistent and recurrent finding.[10] Of note, women more than men tend to have depression as the first episode, suggesting a reason for the higher incidence of suicidal ideation in women compared with men. Further, the polarity of the first episode tends to predict the most common episode phases in the future. Thus, early depression predicts recurrent depression and high-risk phases for suicide attempts.

Rapid Cycling

Several researchers have identified rapid cycling as a high-risk factor for suicide behaviors[36]; however, studies observing this variable are limited.

BIPOLAR DISORDER, SUICIDE, AND MEDICATIONS
Do Antidepressants Increase the Risk of Suicide?

In the early 2000s, reports began to associate a possible link between suicide in children and adolescents.[44,45] The Food and Drug Administration (FDA) mandated that all antidepressants carry a black box warning of suicidality. Although this initially was for children and adolescents, the warning was extended in 2004 to adults up to age 25 years. Since that time, the FDA has also required manufacturers of antiepileptic drugs (AEDs) to include a warning about increased risk of suicidality in their labeling as well. Thus was created the concept that a particular class of drugs may have suicide-promoting effects.

The use of antidepressants in bipolar disorder already is a controversial practice, yet it remains extremely common. It has been noted that more than one-half of all patients with bipolar disorder have been treated with an antidepressant.[46,47] Expert guidelines repeatedly call for extreme caution in the use of antidepressants. The fact that this medicine, so least recommended by the experts for treatment in bipolar disorder yet most widely used by clinicians, reflects both the large need for treatment and the limited options available.

Do antidepressants then increase the risk of suicide in bipolar disorder? It is known that they are primarily used in bipolar disorder to treat the mood state that is highly associated with increased risk of suicide (depression). It is also known that antidepressants can cause switching of mood states, or induce some type of behavioral activation that may increase risk.[48] Multiple studies in bipolar disorder have repeatedly identified increased risk of suicide behaviors in patients treated with antidepressants.[49–52] Although it is tempting to then to assess all antidepressants as suicide-promoting agents, it should be remembered that suicide and suicide behaviors are complex and multifaceted. Thus, direct associations can be difficult to confirm. McElroy and colleagues[53] reviewed 5 studies that demonstrated increased suicidality with antidepressants in bipolar patients, and noted that the findings in 4 of the 5 studies could potentially be explained by the fact that higher suicidal risk may actually have led to the choice of an antidepressant rather than the reverse. Methodologic difficulties still need to be resolved.[48] Overall, the best available evidence suggests that antidepressant use in bipolar disorder does contribute to suicidal behaviors. In fact, the new onset of suicidal thoughts after introduction of an antidepressant in depressed patients should raise the clinician's suspicion of an underlying bipolar illness.[48,54]

Are Anticonvulsants Associated with Increased Suicidal Behaviors?

In 2005, the FDA began studying the association of suicide behaviors in AEDs. The metaanalysis of 199 randomized placebo-controlled trials of the 11 AEDs showed the adjusted risk estimate for suicidal behavior or ideation was 0.43% for drug patients and 0.24% for placebo. The FDA conducted subanalyses for 3 indication categories: epilepsy, psychiatric conditions, and other conditions. Bipolar disorder was not a separate group, but subsumed in the psychiatric condition group. In this group, the overall risk was 1.51, but the confidence interval was 0.95 to 2.45. Of the 11 drugs that had studies for psychiatric conditions, only carbamazepine and divalproex, the most commonly used AEDs for bipolar disorder, had overall risks of less than 1.[48] In their review, Yerevanian and Choi[48] noted that conclusions about the effects of AEDs on suicidal ideation in bipolar disorder were not possible form the FDA study data. Further, an ad hoc task force of the Commission on Neuropsychobiology of the international League Against Epilepsy issued an expert consensus statements noting that given the large number of studies with conflicting results, it was not possible to determine whether AEDs in general are associate with suicidal behaviors.[55] Studies with divalproex in bipolar disorder have suggested that it does not acutely induce suicidal behaviors, and may actually demonstrate some protective effects against suicidality when compared with no treatment over the long term.[44,56,57]

Is Lithium a Suicide-Protective Medication?

Lithium is the best studied medication in relationship to its effect on suicidal behaviors and the only medication that has convincingly been shown to reduce suicidal risk in bipolar patients. Multiple reviews and metaanalyses have confirmed this finding.[18,48,58–61] Baldessarini and colleagues,[18] reviewing 31 studies, noted that the use of lithium in bipolar treatment was associated with a reduction of suicide completion and attempts by 80% compared with no treatment. Cipriani and colleagues[61] noted that lithium use was associated with a 4- to 5-fold decrease in the risk of completed suicides and deliberate nonfatal self-harm events.

Several researchers have also noted a possible association between reduced suicide rates in municipalities that have higher trace amounts of lithium in their drinking water.[62] This observation may be more significant in men than women.

The mechanism of this antisuicide effect is unclear; however, some have suggested that the need for frequent visits and monitoring required for lithium use may contribute to its effect.[48] Others have noted that it is the long term use of lithium that provides suicide-protective properties.[63,64] Therefore, clinicians should be cautious in expecting antisuicide effects in short-term treatment.

NEUROBIOLOGY OF SUICIDE AND SUICIDE BEHAVIORS
If Medications May Influence Suicide Behaviors, Does This Mean That There Is a Neurobiolgic Mechanism Associated with Suicide?

Biological studies in patients with suicidal behaviors and neurochemical studies in postmortem brains of suicide victims have suggested possible neurobiological changes that may be associated with suicide behaviors,[65] although it is not clear if they are causes, consequences, or comorbidity with suicide. Initial research has focused on serotonergic abnormalities, demonstrated by increases of $5HT_{2A}$ and $5HT_{1A}$ receptors in suicidal patients.[66] Bolstering this association has been the decreased prolactin response to fenfluramine suggesting a decrease in 5HT activity overall.[67] Some researchers have noted that 5HT depletion is associated with increased aggression,[65] which may suggest a possible causal mechanism, though this is not conclusive. Other abnormalities noted include changes in the hypothalamic–pituitary–adrenal axis functioning, possibly increased inflammatory factors, or even changes in immune functioning.[68–70] However, as of yet, associations between neurobiological changes and behaviors cannot be related directly. For example, the change in hypothalamic–pituitary–adrenal axis functioning may be related to the stress phenomenon rather than the suicide behavior. However, further study may be helpful in understanding the cascade of events that must occur, both psychologically and neurobiologically, for a patient to consider or act on self-harm thoughts.

PSYCHOTHERAPY AND SUICIDE IN BIPOLAR DISORDER
What About Psychotherapy?

There has been increasing evidence that certain psychosocial interventions combined with psychopharmacological treatment can significantly improve stabilization in bipolar disorder. Cognitive behavioral therapy, in conjunction with medication management, specifically has been shown to decrease suicide behaviors.[71] However, most of the other therapies being investigated for bipolar disorder treatment (family-focused therapy, interpersonal and social rhythm therapy, group psychoeducation, etc), have focused primarily on outcomes in preventing relapses rather than specific suicide behaviors.[72]

SUMMARY

Suicide behaviors remain a major problem for clinicians treating patients with bipolar disorder because suicide behaviors are so intimately associated with the experience of the illness. The reasons for this are not fully known, but by identifying factors that are associated, such as hopelessness, family history of suicide, stressful life events, depressive/mixed episodes, early onset of illness, and comorbid conditions, we have constructed a model suggesting that genetic predispositions of vulnerability and interpersonal/family-of-origin stress, may predispose to suicidal thinking when combined with acute stressors and active depressive illness.

The greatest hope for preventing suicide is in decreasing the time patients may spend in high-risk, suicide-vulnerable episodes. However, the cycling nature of the bipolar illness makes this a very difficult challenge. There are some medications that may be "suicide-preventive" with long-term use, like lithium, or possibly even valproate. There are some medications that may be "suicide provoking," like the antidepressants for children and young adults. However, fuller recommendations on the use of antidepressants in bipolar disorder remains controversial and literature conflicting. Psychotherapy, combined with medication managements, has shown the potential for improving the overall course of the illness and possibly in decreasing suicidal risk.

REFERENCES

1. World Health Organization. Preventing suicide: a global imperative. 2014. p. 1–92. Available at: http://www.who.int/mental_health/suicide-prevention/world_report_2014/en/. Accessed October 13, 2015.
2. Centers for Disease Control and Prevention (CDC). Web-based injury statistics query and reporting system (WISQARS) 2013. Available at: www.cdc.gov/injury/wisqars/index.html.
3. Kessler RC, Berglund P, Borges G, et al. Trends in suicide ideation, plans, gestures, and attempts in the United States, 1990-1992 to 2001-2003. JAMA 2005; 293:2487–95.
4. Mann JJ, Apter A, Bertolote J, et al. Suicide prevention strategies: a systematic review. JAMA 2005;294(16):2064–74.
5. O'Carroll PW, Berman AL, Maris RW, et al. Beyond the tower of babel: a nomenclature for suicidology. Suicide Life Threat Behav 1996;26(3):237–52.
6. Large M, Smith G, Sharma S, et al. Systematic review and meta-analysis of the clinical factors associated with suicide in psychiatric in-patients. Acta Psychiatr Scand 2011;124:18–29.
7. Baldessarini RJ, Hennen J. Genetics of suicide: an overview. Harv Rev Psychiatry 2004;12:1–13.
8. Pompili M, Gonda X, Serafini G, et al. Epidemiology of suicide in bipolar disorders: a systematic review of the literature. Bipolar Disord 2013;15:457–90.
9. Tondo L, Isacsson G, Baldessarini R. Suicidal behaviour in bipolar disorder: risk and prevention. CNS Drugs 2003;17(7):491–511.
10. Schaffer A, Isometsa ET, Tondo L, et al. International society for bipolar disorders task force on suicide: meta-analyses and meta-regression of correlates of suicide attempts and suicide deaths in bipolar disorder. Bipolar Disord 2015;17(1):1–16.
11. Nordentoft M, Mortensen PB, Pedersen CB. Absolute risk of suicide after first hospital contact in mental disorder. Arch Gen Psychiatry 2011;68(10):1058–64.
12. Ilgen MA, Bohnert AS, Ignacio RV, et al. Psychiatric diagnosis and risk of suicide in veterans. Arch Gen Psychiatry 2010;67:1152–8.
13. Rihmer Z, Kiss K. Bipolar disorders and suicidal behaviour. Bipolar Disord 2002; 4(Suppl 1):21–5.

14. Gonda X, Pompili M, Serafini G, et al. Suicidal behavior in bipolar disorder: epidemiology, characteristics and major risk factors. J Affect Disord 2012;143(1–3):16–26.
15. Chen YW, Dilsaver SC. Lifetime rates of suicide attempts among subjects with bipolar and unipolar disorders relative to subjects with other Axis I disorders. Biol Psychiatry 1996;39(10):896–9.
16. Simon NM, Zalta AK, Otto MW, et al. The association of comorbid anxiety disorders with suicide attempts and suicidal ideation in outpatients with bipolar disorder. J Psychiatr Res 2007;41(3–4):255–64.
17. Schaffer A, Cairney J, Veldhuizen S, et al. A population-based analysis of distinguishers of bipolar disorder from major depressive disorder. J Affect Disord 2010; 125(1–3):103–10.
18. Baldessarini RJ, Tondo L, Davis P, et al. Decreased risk of suicides and attempts during long-term lithium treatment: a meta-analytic review. Bipolar Disord 2006; 8(5 Pt 2):625–39.
19. Neves FS, Malloy-Diniz LF, Romano-Silva MA, et al. Is the serotonin transporter polymorphism (5-HTTLPR) a potential marker for suicidal behavior in bipolar disorder patients? J Affect Disord 2010;125(1–3):98–102.
20. Jamison KR. Suicide and bipolar disorder. J Clin Psychiatry 2000;61(Suppl 9): 47–51.
21. Hawton K, van Heeringen K. Suicide. Lancet 2009;373:1372–81.
22. Mann JJ, Waternaux C, Haas GL, et al. Toward a clinical model of suicidal behavior in psychiatric patients. Am J Psychiatry 1999;156:181–9.
23. Tsai SY, Kuo CJ, Chen CC, et al. Risk factors for completed suicide in bipolar disorder. J Clin Psychiatry 2002;63(6):469–76.
24. Algorta GP, Youngstrom EA, Frazier TW, et al. Suicidality in pediatric bipolar disorder: predictor or outcome of family processes and mixed mood presentation? Bipolar Disord 2011;13(1):76–86.
25. Miklowitz DJ, Chang KD. Prevention of bipolar disorder in at-risk children: theoretical assumptions and empirical foundations. Dev Psychopathol 2008;20(3): 881–97.
26. De Abreu LN, Nery FG, Harkavy-Friedman JM, et al. Suicide attempts are associated with worse quality of life in patients with bipolar disorder type I. Compr Psychiatry 2012;53(2):125–9.
27. Michalak EE, Yatham LN, Lam RW. Quality of life in bipolar disorder: a review of the literature. Health Qual Life Outcomes 2005;15:3–72.
28. Coryell W, Fiedorowicz J, Leon AC, et al. Age of onset and the prospectively observed course of illness in bipolar disorder. J Affect Disord 2013;146(1):34–8.
29. Valtonen HM, Suominen K, Mantere O, et al. Prospective study of risk factors for attempted suicide among patients with bipolar disorder. Bipolar Disord 2006;8(5 Pt 2):576–85.
30. Carra G, Bartoli F, Crocamo C, et al. Attempted suicide in people with co-occurring bipolar and substance use disorders: systematic review and meta-analysis. J Affect Disord 2014;167:125–35.
31. Perroud N, Baud P, Preisig M, et al. Social phobia is associated with suicide attempt history in bipolar inpatients. Bipolar Disord 2007;9(7):713–21.
32. Nakagawa A, Grunebaum MF, Sullivan GM, et al. Comorbid anxiety in bipolar disorder: does it have an independent effect on suicidality? Bipolar Disord 2008; 10(4):530–8.
33. Maser JD, Akiskal HS, Schettler P, et al. Can temperament identify affectively ill patients who engage in lethal or near-lethal suicidal behavior? A 14-year prospective study. Suicide Life Threat Behav 2002;32(1):10–32.

34. Watkins HB, Meyer TD. Is there an empirical link between impulsivity and suicidality in bipolar disorders? A review of the current literature and the potential psychological implications of the relationship. Bipolar Disord 2013;15(5): 542–58.
35. Acosta FJ, Vega D, Torralba L, et al. Hopelessness and suicidal risk in bipolar disorder. A study in clinically nonsyndromal patients. Compr Psychiatry 2012;53(8): 1103–9.
36. Hawton K, Sutton L, Haw C, et al. Suicide and attempted suicide in bipolar disorder: a systematic review of risk factors. J Clin Psychiatry 2005;66(6): 693–704.
37. Cheng D. Higher suicide death rate in Rocky Mountain states and a correlation to altitude. Wilderness Environ Med 2010;21(2):177–8.
38. Huber RS, Coon H, Kim N, et al. Altitude is a risk factor for completed suicide in bipolar disorder. Med Hypotheses 2014;82(3):377–81.
39. Kim N, Mickelson JB, Brenner BE, et al. Altitude, gun ownership, rural areas, and suicide. Am J Psychiatry 2011;168(1):49–54.
40. Holma KM, Haukka J, Suominen K, et al. Differences in incidence of suicide attempts between bipolar I and II disorders and major depressive disorder. Bipolar Disord 2014;16(6):652–61.
41. Goldberg JF, Garno JL, Leon AC, et al. Association of recurrent suicidal ideation with nonremission from acute mixed mania. Am J Psychiatry 1998;155(12): 1753–5.
42. Judd LL, Akiskal HS, Schettler PJ, et al. The long-term natural history of the weekly symptomatic status of bipolar I disorder. Arch Gen Psychiatry 2002; 59(6):530–7.
43. Judd LL, Schettler PJ, Akiskal HS, et al. Long-term symptomatic status of bipolar I vs. bipolar II disorders. Int J Neuropsychopharmacol 2003;6(2):127–37.
44. Gibbons RD, Hur K, Brown CH, et al. Relationship between antiepileptic drugs and suicide attempts in patients with bipolar disorder. Arch Gen Psychiatry 2009;66(12):1354–60.
45. Hammad TA, Laughren T, Racoosin J. Suicidality in pediatric patients treated with antidepressant drugs. Arch Gen Psychiatry 2006;63(3):332–9.
46. Baldessarini RJ, Leahy L, Arcona S, et al. Patterns of psychotropic drug prescription for U.S. patients with diagnoses of bipolar disorders. Psychiatr Serv 2007; 58(1):85–91.
47. Baldessarini R, Henk H, Sklar A, et al. Psychotropic medications for patients with bipolar disorder in the United States: polytherapy and adherence. Psychiatr Serv 2008;59(10):1175–83.
48. Yerevanian BI, Choi YM. Impact of psychotropic drugs on suicide and suicidal behaviors. Bipolar Disord 2013;15:594–621.
49. Marangell LB, Dennehy EB, Wisniewski SR, et al. Case-control analyses of the impact of pharmacotherapy on prospectively observed suicide attempts and completed suicides in bipolar disorder: findings from STEP-BD. J Clin Psychiatry 2008;69(6):916–22.
50. Pacchiarotti I, Valentí M, Colom F, et al. Differential outcome of bipolar patients receiving antidepressant monotherapy versus combination with an antimanic drug. J Affect Disord 2011;129(1–3):321–6.
51. Goldberg JF, Allen MH, Miklowitz DA, et al. Suicidal ideation and pharmacotherapy among STEP-BD patients. Psychiatr Serv 2005;56(12):1534–40.
52. Goldberg JF, Garno JL, Portera L, et al. Correlates of suicidal ideation in dysphoric mania. J Affect Disord 1999;56(1):75–81.

53. McElroy SL, Kotwal R, Kaneria R, et al. Antidepressants and suicidal behavior in bipolar disorder. Bipolar Disord 2006;8(5 Pt 2):596–617.
54. Akiskal HS, Benazzi F, Perugi G, et al. Agitated "unipolar" depression reconceptualized as a depressive mixed state: implications for the antidepressant-suicide controversy. J Affect Disord 2005;85(3):245–58.
55. Mula M, Kanner AM, Schmitz B, et al. Antiepileptic drugs and suicidality: an expert consensus statement from the task force on therapeutic strategies of the ILAE commission on neuropsychobiology. Epilepsia 2013; 54(1):199–203.
56. Yerevanian BI, Koek RJ, Mintz J. Bipolar pharmacotherapy and suicidal behavior. Part I: lithium, divalproex and carbamazepine. J Affect Disord 2007;103(1–3): 5–11.
57. Ahearn EP, Chen P, Hertzberg M, et al. Suicide attempts in veterans with bipolar disorder during treatment with lithium, divalproex, and atypical antipsychotics. J Affect Disord 2013;145(1):77–82.
58. Lewitzka U, Severus E, Bauer R, et al. The suicide prevention effect of lithium: more than 20 years of evidence-a narrative review. Int J Bipolar Disord 2015; 3(1):32.
59. Baldessarini RJ, Tondo L, Hennen J. Lithium treatment and suicide risk in major affective disorders: update and new findings. J Clin Psychiatry 2003;64(Suppl 5):44–52.
60. Tondo L, Hennen J, Baldessarini RJ. Lower suicide risk with long-term lithium treatment in major affective illness: a meta-analysis. Acta Psychiatr Scand 2001;104(3):163–72.
61. Cipriani A, Pretty H, Hawton K, et al. Lithium in the prevention of suicidal behavior and all-cause mortality in patients with mood disorders: a systematic review of randomized trials. Am J Psychiatry 2005;162(10):1805–19.
62. Vita A, De Peri L, Sacchetti E. Lithium in drinking water and suicide prevention: a review of the evidence. Int Clin Psychopharmacol 2015;30(1):1–5.
63. Ahrens B, Müller-Oerlinghausen B, Grof P. Length of lithium treatment needed to eliminate the high mortality of affective disorders. Br J Psychiatry Suppl 1993;21: 27–9.
64. Sani G, Tondo L, Koukopoulos A, et al. Suicide in a large population of former psychiatric inpatients. Psychiatry Clin Neurosci 2011;65(3):286–95.
65. Pandey GN. Biological basis of suicide and suicidal behavior. Bipolar Disord 2013;15:524–41.
66. Pandey GN, Pandey SC, Dwivedi Y, et al. Platelet serotonin-2A receptors: a potential biological marker for suicidal behavior. Am J Psychiatry 1995;152(6): 850–5.
67. Sher L, Oquendo MA, Li S, et al. Prolactin response to fenfluramine administration in patients with unipolar and bipolar depression and healthy controls. Psychoneuroendocrinology 2003;28(4):559–73.
68. Meltzer HY, Perline R, Tricou BJ, et al. Effect of 5-hydroxytryptophan on serum cortisol levels in major affective disorders. II. Relation to suicide, psychosis, and depressive symptoms. Arch Gen Psychiatry 1984;41(4):379–87.
69. Yerevanian BI, Feusner JD, Koek RJ, et al. The dexamethasone suppression test as a predictor of suicidal behavior in unipolar depression. J Affect Disord 2004; 83(2–3):103–8.
70. Steiner J, Bielau H, Brisch R, et al. Immunological aspects in the neurobiology of suicide: elevated microglial density in schizophrenia and depression is associated with suicide. J Psychiatr Res 2008;42(2):151–7.

71. Wasserman D, Rihmer Z, Rujescu D, et al, European Psychiatric Association. The European Psychiatric Association (EPA) guidance on suicide treatment and prevention. Eur Psychiatry 2012;27(2):129–41.

72. Fountoulakis KN, Gonda X, Siamouli M, et al. Psychotherapeutic intervention and suicide risk reduction in bipolar disorder: a review of the evidence. J Affect Disord 2009;113(1–2):21–9.

Bipolar Disorder and Inflammation

Joshua D. Rosenblat, MD, Roger S. McIntyre, MD, FRCPC*

KEYWORDS

- Bipolar depression • Inflammation • Innate immune system • NAC • NSAIDs
- Infliximab • Minocycline • Antiinflammatory

KEY POINTS

- Mounting evidence has suggested that dysfunction of the innate immune system may play a key role in the pathophysiology of bipolar disorder (BD).
- Epidemiologic studies have identified elevated rates of inflammatory medical comorbidities in BD subjects as well as a decreased life expectancy.
- Elevated levels of proinflammatory cytokines centrally and peripherally have been identified in BD and are implicated in the pathophysiology of BD.
- Several biologically plausible mechanisms have been proposed to explain the bidirectional interaction between BD and immune dysfunction.
- The innate immune system is as a novel therapeutic target in BD. Several agents with antiinflammatory properties have shown promise in treating bipolar depression.

INTRODUCTION

Bipolar disorder (BD) is a chronic and disabling mental disorder with significant morbidity and mortality.[1,2] The pathophysiology of BD remains poorly understood. Further, current treatments yield high rates of treatment resistance, particularly with bipolar depression, and are often poorly tolerated.[3] An improved understanding of

Authors' Contributions: All authors contributed to the development of the research hypothesis and scope of the article. J.D. Rosenblat conducted the literature search, qualitative analysis and wrote the initial draft of the article. All authors contributed to the interpretation of the literature and article writing.

Conflicts of Interest: J.D. Rosenblat has no conflicts of interest. R.S. McIntyre has received research grant support from Lundbeck, AstraZeneca, Pfizer, Shire, Otsuka, Bristol-Myers Squibb, National Institute of Mental Health, Stanley Medical Research Institute, Canadian Institutes of Health Research, and The Brain and Behavior Research Foundation. R.S. McIntyre has also received speaker/consultant fees from Lundbeck, Pfizer, AstraZeneca, Elli Lilly, Janssen Ortho, Sunovion, Takeda, Forest, Otsuka, Bristol Myers Squibb and Shire.

Mood Disorder Psychopharmacology Unit, University Health Network, University of Toronto, 399 Bathurst Street, MP 9-325, Toronto, Ontario M5T 2S8, Canada
* Corresponding author.
E-mail address: roger.mcintyre@uhn.ca

psych.theclinics.com

the pathophysiology is thus of great importance to allow for the discovery of novel targets, which may yield improved outcomes in the treatment of BD.[4]

Dysfunction of the innate immune system leading to neuroinflammation has been increasingly implicated in the pathophysiology of numerous psychiatric disorders.[5–8] Interest has grown in the role of inflammation in BD after Horrobin and Lieb[9] (1983) initially hypothesized that immune system modulation may play a role in the effects of lithium in BD. Epidemiologic evidence of increased rates of inflammatory medical comorbidities in BD and vice versa further motivated the investigation of the interaction between BD and inflammation.[6] Currently, mounting evidence strongly supports the hypothesis that alterations in the innate immune–inflammatory system are critical to the pathophysiology of BD.[6,10,11] Innate immune dysfunction has thus been identified as a novel target of treatment of BD with numerous clinical trials of antiinflammatory agents currently underway.[12] As such, targeting immune dysfunction shows promise to be translated from purely a research endeavor to clinical practice in the near future.

The objective of the current review is to summarize succinctly the evidence for the interaction between BD and inflammation in a clinically relevant manner. The relevance of this interaction as it pertains to medical comorbidity and decreased life expectancy in BD is also discussed. A discussion of therapeutic implications, including completed and ongoing clinical trials of antiinflammatory agents, ensues.

METHODS

For this narrative clinical overview, the MEDLINE/PubMed, Embase, Google Scholar and ClinicalTrials.gov databases were searched from inception through June 2015 for published reviews, metaanalyses and primary studies of the relationship between BD and immune dysfunction. Also, randomized controlled trials (RCTs), open-label trials, metaanalyses, and systematic reviews of antiinflammatory agents for the treatment of BD were searched for. Searches terms included various combinations of the following terms: Bipolar disorder (BD), bipolar depression, novel targets, inflammation, immune dysfunction, infliximab, cytokines, interleukin (IL), IL-1B, IL-6, tumor necrosis factor alpha (TNF-α), anti–TNF-α, nonsteroidal antiinflammatory drugs, celecoxib, acetylsalicylic acid, omega-3 polyunsaturated fatty acid (omega-3s), curcumin, oxidative stress, reactive oxygen species, hypothalamic–pituitary–adrenal axis, cortisol, metabolic syndrome, diabetes, cardiovascular disease, autoimmune disease, systemic lupus erythematosus, rheumatoid arthritis, psoriasis, Guillain-Barre syndrome, Crohn's disease, ulcerative colitis, and inflammatory bowel disease. Reference lists from included papers were also manually searched for additional pertinent references.

RESULTS
Bipolar Disorder, Inflammation, and Medical Comorbidity

BD has been associated with significantly increased rates of several medical comorbidities.[13–20] Further, BD is associated with a significantly decreased life expectancy secondary to increased rates of diabetes, cardiovascular disease, and all-cause mortality.[21,22] Factors contributing to the foregoing increased rate of medical comorbidity are likely multidimensional; however, immune dysfunction has been proposed as a significant factor.[6,22] Indeed, several of the medical comorbidities of BD are inflammatory in nature.[6]

Inflammatory comorbidities that have been associated with BD include inflammatory bowel disease, systemic lupus erythematosus, autoimmune thyroiditis, psoriasis,

Guillain-Barré syndrome, autoimmune hepatitis, multiple sclerosis, migraines, rheumatoid arthritis, obesity, atherosclerosis, and type II diabetes mellitus, as shown by epidemiologic studies.[15,17,23–31] Of note, aside from diagnosed inflammatory medical comorbidities, several other factors may result in inflammation in BD, including but not limited to undiagnosed inflammatory medical comorbidities, history of early childhood adversity, chronic oxidative stress, a dysfunctional gut microbiota, and low-grade, idiopathic systemic inflammation.[32–36]

The direction of causation has yet to be established; however, the temporal relationship of BD and inflammatory conditions suggests that the interaction between BD, inflammation, and medical comorbidities is likely bidirectional.[17] Inflammation may be a common cause to both BD and medical comorbidity. Alternatively, medical comorbidity may induce an inflammatory state, thus increasing the risk of developing BD or vice versa. Indeed, BD may predate an inflammatory comorbidity, the comorbidity may predate the onset of BD, or both may have a similar time of onset. Therefore, the direction of causality remains unclear.[6]

Taken together, mounting evidence suggests a significant association between BD and inflammatory comorbidities. The identified association has yet to be established as causal; however, the available evidence suggests that the relationship is bidirectional. Identifying and targeting this interaction with novel treatments might therefore allow for the simultaneous treatment of BD and the medical comorbidity. Moreover, if inflammation is a pathophysiologic nexus between BD and medical comorbidity, targeting inflammation may potentially provide disease-modifying effects for both disease processes.[10] In keeping with this hypothesis, immune dysfunction in BD may be a major factor contributing to the observed decreased life expectancy in BD.[22]

Bipolar Disorder and Cytokine Levels

A central method for determining the association between BD and immune dysfunction has been the measurement of peripheral (eg, in blood) and central (eg, in the cerebral spinal fluid) markers of inflammation. Cytokine levels in BD subjects have been measured in numerous studies to determine the presence and strength of the association between inflammation and BD, as well as to identify the key elements of the immune system that are perturbed.[11,37–40]

The majority of these cytokine studies measure peripheral cytokine levels, although relatively few studies have investigated central cytokine levels in BD.[11,37–40] Although central levels may be more relevant because they may be more directly indicative of neuroinflammation, the safety and invasiveness of venipuncture compared with lumbar puncture often dictates the preferential use of protocols measuring peripheral cytokine level. Nevertheless, numerous studies have correlated peripheral and central cytokine levels.[11,37–40]

Peripheral cytokines may traverse the blood–brain barrier through leaky regions of the choroid plexus as well via active transport.[41] In addition, a recent study showed functional lymphatic vessels lining the dural sinuses in an animal model.[42] This breakthrough discovery contradicted the conventional thinking that the central nervous system was devoid of a classical lymphatic drainage system. The presence of lymphatic vessels in the central nervous system thus provides an additional potential avenue for cytokines to be transported to and from the brain. Taken together, peripheral cytokine levels may strongly affect central cytokine levels and also provide as a reasonable marker of neuroinflammation.

Determining cytokine level changes may provide great insight into the mechanistic underpinnings of how immune dysfunction may be affecting brain function and mood disorder pathophysiology. Several studies have now shown proinflammatory cytokines to be elevated during periods of depression, mania, and euthymia, indicative of a chronic, low-grade inflammatory state.[37,39,43–47] More specifically, serum levels of proinflammatory molecules IL-4, TNF-α, soluble IL-2 receptor, IL-1β, IL-6, soluble receptor of TNF-alpha type 1 (STNFR1), and C-reactive protein (CRP) are increased in BD patients compared with healthy controls.[37,39,43–47]

Of note, several studies suggest that cytokine levels may vary depending on mood state (**Fig. 1**). During periods of euthymia, sTNFR1 is the only consistently increased inflammatory marker.[37,38,43] During manic episodes, serum levels of IL-6, TNF-α, sTNFR1, IL-RA, CXCL10, CXCL11, and IL-4 have been shown to be increased.[37,38,48,49] During depressive episodes, serum levels of sTNFR1 and CXCL10 are increased.[37,48] Only a limited number of studies have investigated cytokine levels of BD during depressive episodes; however, more robust cytokine studies evaluating individuals experiencing a major depressive episode (MDE) as part of major depressive disorder have demonstrated elevation in serum levels of TNF-α, IL-6, and IL-1β.[5,50–52]

Taken together, these results suggest that BD is associated with a proinflammatory state. More specifically, the cytokine profile indicates dysfunction of the innate immune system. Several studies have suggested variability in cytokine levels depending on mood state. These results suggest that BD is associated with chronic low-grade inflammation (eg, even during periods of euthymia) with periods of increased inflammation that are, at times, associated with mood episodes (eg, mania or depression). Notably, however, the majority of studies are cross-sectional in nature, and report

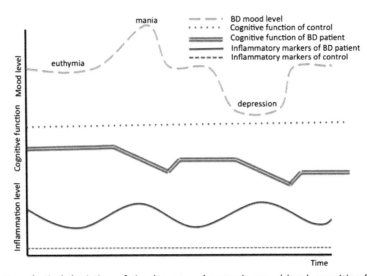

Fig. 1. Hypothetical depiction of simultaneous changes in mood level, cognitive function, and inflammatory cytokine levels. Cytokine levels are elevated chronically and may increase during both manic and depressive episodes. Based on the current evidence, we hypothesize that these increased levels of cytokines and mood episodes may also be associated with a decline in cognitive function. With resolution of mood episodes, some cognitive function may be restored; however, evidence suggests that cognitive function is still lower than healthy controls, even during euthymic periods. Each mood episode may induce the neuroprogression of disease, facilitating decreased neural circuit function in key brain regions subserving cognition. With each stepwise decline in cognition, a new lower baseline may be established. This proposed decline in cognition secondary to inflammation and mood episodes in bipolar disorder (BD) has yet to be fully established; however, it presents as a testable hypothesis of interest.

the mood state of the subject at the time of blood sampling. The cross-sectional nature of these studies may be misleading; for example, if a patient is euthymic on the day of the blood draw, however, the day before was manic, the cytokine levels may be still influenced by the previous day's levels. Therefore, the variability of cytokine levels relative to mood state remains unclear. Future studies are needed to measure longitudinally cytokine levels within the same group of BD subjects to see if and how cytokine levels are altered during mood episodes.

Cytokine Levels and Cognitive Dysfunction in Bipolar Disorder

The previously discussed cytokine studies focused on cytokine levels as related to specific mood states (eg, euthymic, depressed, or manic). Recently, interest has also grown in the relationship between cytokine levels and cognitive dysfunction in BD.[53] Cognitive dysfunction has become a key therapeutic target of interest because it has been shown to be a strong determinant of functional impairment in BD.[53–57] Further, cognitive dysfunction is often still present during periods of remission and is affected minimally by current conventional mood-stabilizing treatments.[58] Therefore, a greater understanding of cognitive dysfunction in BD is needed to yield new therapeutic targets and improved outcomes. Inflammation has been suggested as a potential target of interest.[53]

Several studies have reported that elevated levels of proinflammatory cytokines in BD are associated with poorer cognitive function.[59–64] Results from these studies indicate that cognitive dysfunction is highly associated with elevated levels of proinflammatory markers YKL40, IL-6, sCD40L, IL-1Ra, CRP, and TNF-α. Therefore, dysfunction of the innate immune system may also be associated with progressive worsening of cognitive dysfunction in BD (see **Fig. 1**).

Proposed Pathophysiologic Mechanism

Dysfunction of the innate immune system may have deleterious effects on mood and cognition in BD subjects through numerous pathophysiologic pathways.[5] Preclinical and clinical studies have found, and continue to elucidate, potential pathophysiologic pathways.[5,8,65,66] These pathways provide biologically plausible mechanisms whereby neuroinflammation may affect the structure and function of key brain regions subserving mood and cognition.[67]

The direct effect of cytokines on monoamine levels serves as one key mechanism whereby inflammation may affect mood and cognition. The proinflammatory cytokines TNF-α, IL-2, and IL-6 have been shown to directly alter monoamine levels.[68] IL-2 and interferon increase the enzymatic activity of indolamine 2,3-dioxygenase, thus increasing the breakdown of tryptophan to depressogenic tryptophan catabolites.[5,66] Depletion of tryptophan leading to decreased levels of serotonin production and release has long been recognized as an important potential mechanism subserving affective and cognitive dysfunction.[69,70] Serotonin levels may be further modulated through the IL-6– and TNF-α–dependent breakdown of serotonin to 5-hydroxyindoleacetic acid.[71,72] Taken together, proinflammatory cytokines may induce both mood and cognitive dysfunction by promoting depletion of tryptophan, breakdown of serotonin, and production of depressogenic tryptophan to depressogenic tryptophan catabolites.

Another key mechanism that has been elucidated is the overactivation of microglia, the macrophages of the central nervous system, in BD.[65] Microglia, under physiologic conditions, perform an important role in neuroplasticity, facilitating neural network pruning via inducing apoptosis of neurons and neural pathways that are not being frequently used.[73,74] Pruning of these pathways is vital to maintenance and growth of more important (eg, more frequently used) neural pathways.[74] Under hyperinflammatory, pathologic conditions, however, microglia may be overactive, aberrantly destroying important neural pathways.[65,75]

The microglial hypothesis of mood disorders suggests that microglia may be overactivated in key brain regions subserving mood and cognition (eg, the prefrontal cortex, amygdala, hippocampus, insula, and anterior cingulate cortex) in BD subjects.[65,75] In support of this hypothesis, Haarman and colleagues[76] found overactivation of microglia in the right hippocampus of BD subjects compared with healthy controls as shown by PET imaging using a marker of microglial activation. Also of note, Setiawan and colleagues[77] in 2015 showed increased microglial activation in the anterior cingulate cortex, prefrontal cortex, and insula in subjects with major depressive disorder with a current MDE compared with healthy controls, using a similar PET imaging technique. Post mortem studies of BD subjects compared with healthy controls have also shown increased markers of inflammation and microglial activation in the prefrontal cortex, an essential area for affective regulation, executive function, attention, and cognitive control.[78,79]

Overactive microglia also create a positive feedforward loop, activated microglia release cytokines, which further increase inflammation, and further recruitment and activation of microglia.[65,73] The release of cytokines, notably TNF-α, by activated microglia further perpetuate the previously discussed monoamine changes, which may alter mood and cognition. The overactivation of microglia also increases local oxidative stress, further damaging neural circuitry in key brain regions subserving mood and cognition.[65,80]

Another key mechanism whereby inflammation may induce mood dysfunction in BD is hypothalamic–pituitary–adrenal axis dysregulation. Increased levels of proinflammatory cytokines, interferon, TNF-α, and IL-6 upregulate hypothalamic–pituitary–adrenal axis activity, thereby increasing systemic cortisol levels leading to hypercortisolemia.[81–83] Increased cortisol levels may potently alter mood; indeed, induction of both mania and depression via increased levels of exogenous or endogenous steroids has been well-documented.[84] Increased levels of cortisol also increase the activity of hepatic tryptophan 2,3-dioxygenase activity, thereby increasing the breakdown of tryptophan to tryptophan to depressogenic tryptophan catabolites.[85,86]

In addition, increased levels of inflammatory cytokines decrease glucocorticoid receptor synthesis, transport, and sensitivity in the hypothalamus and pituitary.[87,88] Therefore, the negative feedback loop, which usually downregulates cortisol production, is disabled, leading to chronically increased levels of cortisol.[87,88] Further, impaired cortisol suppression itself has long been recognized as a strong predictor of mood disorders.[89,90]

Therapeutic Implications

Currently, psychopharmacologic management of BD is associated with high rates of treatment resistance, particularly with bipolar depression.[3] Given the replicated and convergent evidence implicating inflammation in the pathophysiology of BD, the immune system presents as a novel target of treatment, which may provide hope for improved outcomes and tolerability.[12] Several studies have sought to determine whether antiinflammatory agents are capable of mitigating depressive symptoms in adults with bipolar depression.[12] For example, clinical trials of N-acetyl-cysteine (NAC),[91,92] nonsteroidal antiinflammatory drugs,[93,94] omega-3 polyunsaturated fatty acids (omega-3s),[95–99] pioglitazone,[100] and minocycline[101] have been conducted. Also of note, lithium, one of the oldest and most effective treatments of bipolar depression, has potent antiinflammatory effects.[9]

NAC, an antiinflammatory and antioxidant agent, is perhaps the most promising antiinflammatory agent that has been assessed in the adjunctive treatment of BD.[91,92] In a large placebo-controlled, RCT, adjunctive NAC was shown to lower depression scores throughout the trial with a statistically significant difference compared with the placebo group by the primary endpoint of 24 weeks.[91] Additionally, a post hoc analysis of 17 patients from this sample who met criteria for a current MDE at baseline, revealed that 8 of the 10 participants in the NAC group demonstrated a response with a 50% reduction in Montgomery–Åsberg Depression Rating Scale during the trial compared with only 1 participant in the placebo group.[102] An 8-week open-label trial of NAC also showed a significant reduction in depressive symptoms in BD subjects[103]; however, during a subsequent 24-week RCT phase of the same sample, there was minimal further change in depression severity with scores remaining low in both groups.[92] Of note, Soares and colleagues are currently conducting a phase II, double-blind RCT of aspirin and NAC as adjunctive treatment for BD (NCT01797575).

Several RCTs have also been conducted evaluating the effects of adjunctive omega-3s, a naturally occurring and well-tolerated antiinflammatory agent.[104] Results have been mixed with several trials showing an antidepressant effect in BD[95,98] and others reporting no significant difference compared with conventional therapy alone.[96,97,99] In a recent metaanalysis, a moderate antidepressant effect of adjunctive omega-3 in BD was found compared with conventional therapy alone.[104]

Adjunctive nonsteroidal antiinflammatory drugs have also been evaluated for relief of depressive symptoms in BD. In 2008, Nery and colleagues[93] assessed adjunctive celecoxib in BD patients in a current depressive or mixed episode. In this study, adjunctive celecoxib lowered Hamilton Rating Scale for Depression by week 1; however, the primary outcome was negative because the change in depression severity converged with the placebo group by the end of week 6. Saroukhani and colleagues[94] in 2013 assessed the effect of adjunctive aspirin in male BD patients and found no difference between treatment groups by the end of the 6-week RCT. Two additional trials assessing celecoxib (NCT01479829) and aspirin (NCT01797575) as adjunctive treatments for BD are currently underway.

Pioglitazone, a peroxisome proliferator activated receptor-gamma agonist with potent antiinflammatory and antihyperglycemic effects, has also been investigated in the treatment of BD.[100] In a 6-week, double-blind RCT in BD patients with a current MDE, a significant decrease in depressive symptom severity was found.[100] In addition, in an open-label trial of BD patients with comorbid metabolic dysfunction, adjunctive pioglitazone treatment was associated with a decrease in depressive symptoms after 8 weeks of treatment.[105] Also of interest, in this open-label trial, higher baseline levels of IL-6 were associated with a greater decrease in depression severity.

The effect of minocycline, a tetracyclic antibiotic with antiinflammatory, antioxidant, and with neuroprotective properties, has also been of interest in BD.[106] Although no clinical trials assessing the effects of minocycline for BD have been published, 3 clinical trials are currently underway (NCT01403662, NCT01514422, NCT01429272).

TNF-α inhibitors have also been of interest in the treatment of BD. One key RCT assessed infliximab in treatment resistant depression (including BD and major depressive disorder subjects in their sample). Although the antidepressant effect was negative for this study overall, a significant antidepressant effect was observed for a subgroup of patients, namely, those with increased levels of serum CRP and TNF-α.[107] The results of this trial were of particular interest because they suggested that stratification using inflammatory biomarkers might help to determine which patients may benefit from antiinflammatory therapies. Currently, a 12-week, multisite, double-blind RCT evaluating the efficacy, safety, and tolerability of adjunctive inflix-imab for the treatment of BD subjects with and elevated serum CRP is currently underway (NCT02363738).

Taken together, several well-tolerated, antiinflammatory agents have been investigated showing promising results for decreasing the depressive symptoms of bipolar depression without inducing manic switches. These findings add further merit to targeting the immune system in the treatment of BD. Of the agents discussed, adjunctive NAC seems to have the greatest evidence for an antidepressant effect in BD. Other antiinflammatory agents require additional research to establish their safety and efficacy in the treatment of bipolar depression.

SUMMARY

Dysfunction of the innate immune system seems to be strongly associated with BD. Elevated levels of proinflammatory cytokines have been associated with BD; this finding has been replicated in several studies and metaanalyses.[38,48] In addition, inflammation seems to be a pathophysiologic nexus facilitating the interaction between BD and the increased coprevalence of medical comorbidity.[6] This increased prevalence of medical comorbidity secondary to inflammation is of particular relevance given the high level of morbidity and decreased life expectancy owing to the all-cause mortality associated with BD.[22] Given the role of inflammation in the pathophysiology of BD, the innate immune system presents as a novel target of treatment. Several clinical trials of adjunctive agents with antiinflammatory properties are showing antidepressant effects in BD.[12] Adjunctive NAC presents with particularly promising results for a moderate antidepressant effect.[91] Ongoing clinical trials of minocycline and infliximab for bipolar depression are also of particular interest. Future clinical trials may benefit from stratifying patients based on inflammatory status (eg, specifically assessing the effect of antiinflammatory agents in BD subjects with increased inflammatory markers). Taken together, targeting the innate immune system presents as a promising new strategy in the treatment of BD that may have clinical implications in the near future; however, further studies are still required to determine the role of antiinflammatory agents in the treatment of BD.

REFERENCES

1. Kupfer DJ. The increasing medical burden in bipolar disorder. JAMA 2005;293:2528–30.
2. Fagiolini A, Forgione R, Maccari M, et al. Prevalence, chronicity, burden and borders of bipolar disorder. J Affect Disord 2013;148:161–9.
3. Gitlin M. Treatment-resistant bipolar disorder. Mol Psychiatry 2006;11:227–40.
4. McIntyre RS. A vision for drug discovery and development: novel targets and multilateral partnerships. Adv Ther 2014;31:245–6.
5. Rosenblat JD, Cha DS, Mansur RB, et al. Inflamed moods: a review of the interactions between inflammation and mood disorders. Prog NeuroPsychopharmacol Biol Psychiatry 2014;53:23–34.
6. Rosenblat JD, McIntyre RS. Are medical comorbid conditions of bipolar disorder due to immune dysfunction? Acta Psychiatr Scand 2015;132(3):180–91.
7. Miller AH, Haroon E, Raison CL, et al. Cytokine targets in the brain: impact on neurotransmitters and neurocircuits. Depress Anxiety 2013;30:297–306.
8. Raison CL, Miller AH. Malaise, melancholia and madness: the evolutionary legacy of an inflammatory bias. Brain Behav Immun 2013;31:1–8.

 9. Horrobin DF, Lieb J. A biochemical basis for the actions of lithium on behaviour and on immunity: relapsing and remitting disorders of inflammation and immunity such as multiple sclerosis or recurrent herpes as manic-depression of the immune system. Med Hypotheses 1981;7:891–905.
10. Goldstein BI, Kemp DE, Soczynska JK, et al. Inflammation and the phenomenology, pathophysiology, comorbidity, and treatment of bipolar disorder: a systematic review of the literature. J Clin Psychiatry 2009;70:1078–90.
11. Munkholm K, Brauner JV, Kessing LV, et al. Cytokines in bipolar disorder vs. healthy control subjects: a systematic review and meta-analysis. J Psychiatr Res 2013;47:1119–33.
12. Ayorech Z, Tracy DK, Baumeister D, et al. Taking the fuel out of the fire: evidence for the use of anti-inflammatory agents in the treatment of bipolar disorders. J Affect Disord 2015;174:467–78.
13. Klumpers UM, Boom K, Janssen FM, et al. Cardiovascular risk factors in outpatients with bipolar disorder. Pharmacopsychiatry 2004;37:211–6.
14. McIntyre RS, Danilewitz M, Liauw SS, et al. Bipolar disorder and metabolic syndrome: an international perspective. J Affect Disord 2010;126:366–87.
15. McIntyre RS, Konarski JZ, Misener VL, et al. Bipolar disorder and diabetes mellitus: epidemiology, etiology, and treatment implications. Ann Clin Psychiatry 2005;17:83–93.
16. Osby U, Brandt L, Correia N, et al. Excess mortality in bipolar and unipolar disorder in Sweden. Arch Gen Psychiatry 2001;58:844–50.
17. Perugi G, Quaranta G, Belletti S, et al. General medical conditions in 347 bipolar disorder patients: Clinical correlates of metabolic and autoimmune-allergic diseases. J Affect Disord 2014;170C:95–103.
18. Swartz HA, Fagiolini A. Cardiovascular disease and bipolar disorder: risk and clinical implications. J Clin Psychiatry 2012;73:1563–5.
19. Vancampfort D, Vansteelandt K, Correll CU, et al. Metabolic syndrome and metabolic abnormalities in bipolar disorder: a meta-analysis of prevalence rates and moderators. Am J Psychiatry 2013;170:265–74.
20. Young AH, Grunze H. Physical health of patients with bipolar disorder. Acta Psychiatr Scand Suppl 2013;442:3–10.
21. Kessing LV, Vradi E, Andersen PK. Life expectancy in bipolar disorder. Bipolar Disord 2015;17(5):543–8.
22. Kessing LV, Vradi E, McIntyre RS, et al. Causes of decreased life expectancy over the life span in bipolar disorder. J Affect Disord 2015;180:142–7.
23. Eaton WW, Pedersen MG, Nielsen PR, et al. Autoimmune diseases, bipolar disorder, and non-affective psychosis. Bipolar Disord 2010;12:638–46.
24. Bachen EA, Chesney MA, Criswell LA. Prevalence of mood and anxiety disorders in women with systemic lupus erythematosus. Arthritis Rheum 2009;61:822–9.
25. Kupka RW, Nolen WA, Post RM, et al. High rate of autoimmune thyroiditis in bipolar disorder: lack of association with lithium exposure. Biol Psychiatry 2002;51:305–11.
26. Hsu CC, Chen SC, Liu CJ, et al. Rheumatoid arthritis and the risk of bipolar disorder: a nationwide population-based study. PLoS One 2014;9:e107512.
27. Edwards LJ, Constantinescu CS. A prospective study of conditions associated with multiple sclerosis in a cohort of 658 consecutive outpatients attending a multiple sclerosis clinic. Mult Scler 2004;10:575–81.
28. Calkin C, van de Velde C, Ruzickova M, et al. Can body mass index help predict outcome in patients with bipolar disorder? Bipolar Disord 2009;11:650–6.

29. Lilliker SL. Prevalence of diabetes in a manic-depressive population. Compr Psychiatry 1980;21:270–5.
30. Cassidy F, Ahearn E, Carroll BJ. Elevated frequency of diabetes mellitus in hospitalized manic-depressive patients. Am J Psychiatry 1999;156:1417–20.
31. Han C, Lofland JH, Zhao N, et al. Increased prevalence of psychiatric disorders and health care-associated costs among patients with moderate-to-severe psoriasis. J Drugs Dermatol 2011;10:843–50.
32. Bercik P. The microbiota-gut-brain axis: learning from intestinal bacteria? Gut 2011;60:288–9.
33. Cryan JF, Dinan TG. Mind-altering microorganisms: the impact of the gut microbiota on brain and behaviour. Nat Rev Neurosci 2012;13:701–12.
34. Brietzke E, Mansur RB, Soczynska JK, et al. Towards a multifactorial approach for prediction of bipolar disorder in at risk populations. J Affect Disord 2012;140:82–91.
35. Post RM, Altshuler LL, Leverich GS, et al. Role of childhood adversity in the development of medical co-morbidities associated with bipolar disorder. J Affect Disord 2013;147:288–94.
36. Fagundes CP, Glaser R, Kiecolt-Glaser JK. Stressful early life experiences and immune dysregulation across the lifespan. Brain Behav Immun 2013;27:8–12.
37. Barbosa IG, Bauer ME, Machado-Vieira R, et al. Cytokines in bipolar disorder: paving the way for neuroprogression. Neural Plast 2014;2014:360481.
38. Barbosa IG, Rocha NP, Bauer ME, et al. Chemokines in bipolar disorder: trait or state? Eur Arch Psychiatry Clin Neurosci 2013;263:159–65.
39. Modabbernia A, Taslimi S, Brietzke E, et al. Cytokine alterations in bipolar disorder: a meta-analysis of 30 studies. Biol Psychiatry 2013;74:15–25.
40. Munkholm K, Vinberg M, Vedel Kessing L. Cytokines in bipolar disorder: a systematic review and meta-analysis. J Affect Disord 2013;144:16–27.
41. Weller RO, Engelhardt B, Phillips MJ. Lymphocyte targeting of the central nervous system: a review of afferent and efferent CNS-immune pathways. Brain Pathol 1996;6:275–88.
42. Louveau A, Smirnov I, Keyes TJ, et al. Structural and functional features of central nervous system lymphatic vessels. Nature 2015;523:337–41.
43. Brietzke E, Kauer-Sant'Anna M, Teixeira AL, et al. Abnormalities in serum chemokine levels in euthymic patients with bipolar disorder. Brain Behav Immun 2009;23:1079–82.
44. Brietzke E, Stertz L, Fernandes BS, et al. Comparison of cytokine levels in depressed, manic and euthymic patients with bipolar disorder. J Affect Disord 2009;116:214–7.
45. Breunis MN, Kupka RW, Nolen WA, et al. High numbers of circulating activated T cells and raised levels of serum IL-2 receptor in bipolar disorder. Biol Psychiatry 2003;53:157–65.
46. Drexhage RC, Hoogenboezem TH, Versnel MA, et al. The activation of monocyte and T cell networks in patients with bipolar disorder. Brain Behav Immun 2011;25:1206–13.
47. O'Brien SM, Scully P, Scott LV, et al. Cytokine profiles in bipolar affective disorder: focus on acutely ill patients. J Affect Disord 2006;90:263–7.
48. Barbosa IG, Machado-Vieira R, Soares JC, et al. The immunology of bipolar disorder. Neuroimmunomodulation 2014;21:117–22.
49. Liu HC, Yang YY, Chou YM, et al. Immunologic variables in acute mania of bipolar disorder. J Neuroimmunol 2004;150:116–22.

50. Dantzer R, O'Connor JC, Freund GG, et al. From inflammation to sickness and depression: when the immune system subjugates the brain. Nat Rev Neurosci 2008;9:46–56.
51. Eller T, Vasar V, Shlik J, et al. The role of IL-2 and soluble IL-2R in depression and antidepressant response. Curr Opin Investig Drugs 2009;10:638–43.
52. Felger JC, Lotrich FE. Inflammatory cytokines in depression: neurobiological mechanisms and therapeutic implications. Neuroscience 2013;246:199–229.
53. Bauer IE, Pascoe MC, Wollenhaupt-Aguiar B, et al. Inflammatory mediators of cognitive impairment in bipolar disorder. J Psychiatr Res 2014;56:18–27.
54. Tse S, Chan S, Ng KL, et al. Meta-analysis of predictors of favorable employment outcomes among individuals with bipolar disorder. Bipolar Disord 2014; 16:217–29.
55. Green MF. Cognitive impairment and functional outcome in schizophrenia and bipolar disorder. J Clin Psychiatry 2006;67(Suppl 9):3–8 [discussion: 36–42].
56. Daniel BD, Montali A, Gerra ML, et al. Cognitive impairment and its associations with the path of illness in affective disorders: a comparison between patients with bipolar and unipolar depression in remission. J Psychiatr Pract 2013;19: 275–87.
57. Godard J, Baruch P, Grondin S, et al. Psychosocial and neurocognitive functioning in unipolar and bipolar depression: a 12-month prospective study. Psychiatry Res 2012;196:145–53.
58. Bourne C, Aydemir O, Balanza-Martinez V, et al. Neuropsychological testing of cognitive impairment in euthymic bipolar disorder: an individual patient data meta-analysis. Acta Psychiatr Scand 2013;128:149–62.
59. Lotrich FE, Butters MA, Aizenstein H, et al. The relationship between interleukin-1 receptor antagonist and cognitive function in older adults with bipolar disorder. Int J Geriatr Psychiatry 2014;29:635–44.
60. Hamdani N, Daban-Huard C, Lajnef M, et al. Cognitive deterioration among bipolar disorder patients infected by Toxoplasma gondii is correlated to interleukin 6 levels. J Affect Disord 2015;179:161–6.
61. Hope S, Hoseth E, Dieset I, et al. Inflammatory markers are associated with general cognitive abilities in schizophrenia and bipolar disorder patients and healthy controls. Schizophr Res 2015;165(2–3):188–94.
62. Dickerson F, Stallings C, Origoni A, et al. Elevated C-reactive protein and cognitive deficits in individuals with bipolar disorder. J Affect Disord 2013;150:456–9.
63. Doganavsargil-Baysal O, Cinemre B, Aksoy UM, et al. Levels of TNF-alpha, soluble TNF receptors (sTNFR1, sTNFR2), and cognition in bipolar disorder. Hum Psychopharmacol 2013;28:160–7.
64. Barbosa IG, Rocha NP, Huguet RB, et al. Executive dysfunction in euthymic bipolar disorder patients and its association with plasma biomarkers. J Affect Disord 2012;137:151–5.
65. Stertz L, Magalhaes PV, Kapczinski F. Is bipolar disorder an inflammatory condition? The relevance of microglial activation. Curr Opin Psychiatry 2013;26:19–26.
66. Dunn AJ, Swiergiel AH, de Beaurepaire R. Cytokines as mediators of depression: what can we learn from animal studies? Neurosci Biobehav Rev 2005; 29:891–909.
67. McNamara RK, Lotrich FE. Elevated immune-inflammatory signaling in mood disorders: a new therapeutic target? Expert Rev Neurother 2012;12:1143–61.
68. Capuron L, Neurauter G, Musselman DL, et al. Interferon-alpha-induced changes in tryptophan metabolism. relationship to depression and paroxetine treatment. Biol Psychiatry 2003;54:906–14.

69. Arango V, Underwood MD, Mann JJ. Serotonin brain circuits involved in major depression and suicide. Prog Brain Res 2002;136:443–53.
70. Buhot MC, Martin S, Segu L. Role of serotonin in memory impairment. Ann Med 2000;32:210–21.
71. Wang J, Dunn AJ. Mouse interleukin-6 stimulates the HPA axis and increases brain tryptophan and serotonin metabolism. Neurochem Int 1998;33:143–54.
72. Zhang J, Terreni L, De Simoni MG, et al. Peripheral interleukin-6 administration increases extracellular concentrations of serotonin and the evoked release of serotonin in the rat striatum. Neurochem Int 2001;38:303–8.
73. Ekdahl CT. Microglial activation - tuning and pruning adult neurogenesis. Front Pharmacol 2012;3:41.
74. Harry GJ, Kraft AD. Microglia in the developing brain: a potential target with life-time effects. Neurotoxicology 2012;33:191–206.
75. Frick LR, Williams K, Pittenger C. Microglial dysregulation in psychiatric disease. Clin Dev Immunol 2013;2013:608654.
76. Haarman BC, Riemersma-Van der Lek RF, de Groot JC, et al. Neuroinflammation in bipolar disorder - A [(11)C]-(R)-PK11195 positron emission tomography study. Brain Behav Immun 2014;40:219–25.
77. Setiawan E, Wilson AA, Mizrahi R, et al. Role of translocator protein density, a marker of neuroinflammation, in the brain during major depressive episodes. JAMA Psychiatry 2015;72:268–75.
78. Rao JS, Harry GJ, Rapoport SI, et al. Increased excitotoxicity and neuroinflammatory markers in postmortem frontal cortex from bipolar disorder patients. Mol Psychiatry 2010;15:384–92.
79. Bezchlibnyk YB, Wang JF, McQueen GM, et al. Gene expression differences in bipolar disorder revealed by cDNA array analysis of post-mortem frontal cortex. J Neurochem 2001;79:826–34.
80. Kraft AD, Harry GJ. Features of microglia and neuroinflammation relevant to environmental exposure and neurotoxicity. Int J Environ Res Public Health 2011;8:2980–3018.
81. Beishuizen A, Thijs LG. Endotoxin and the hypothalamo-pituitary-adrenal (HPA) axis. J Endotoxin Res 2003;9:3–24.
82. Harrison NA, Brydon L, Walker C, et al. Inflammation causes mood changes through alterations in subgenual cingulate activity and mesolimbic connectivity. Biol Psychiatry 2009;66:407–14.
83. Wright CE, Strike PC, Brydon L, et al. Acute inflammation and negative mood: mediation by cytokine activation. Brain Behav Immun 2005;19:345–50.
84. Murphy BE. Steroids and depression. J Steroid Biochem Mol Biol 1991;38:537–59.
85. Hoes MJ, Sijben N. The clinical significance of disordered renal excretion of xanthurenic acid in depressive patients. Psychopharmacology 1981;75:346–9.
86. Maes M, Leonard BE, Myint AM, et al. The new '5-HT' hypothesis of depression: cell-mediated immune activation induces indoleamine 2,3-dioxygenase, which leads to lower plasma tryptophan and an increased synthesis of detrimental tryptophan catabolites (TRYCATs), both of which contribute to the onset of depression. Prog Neuro-Psychopharmacology Biol Psychiatry 2011;35:702–21.
87. Pace TW, Miller AH. Cytokines and glucocorticoid receptor signaling. Relevance to major depression. Ann N Y Acad Sci 2009;1179:86–105.
88. Turnbull AV, Rivier CL. Regulation of the hypothalamic-pituitary-adrenal axis by cytokines: actions and mechanisms of action. Physiol Rev 1999;79:1–71.
89. Cowen PJ. Not fade away: the HPA axis and depression. Psychol Med 2010;40:1–4.

90. Rush AJ, Giles DE, Schlesser MA, et al. The dexamethasone suppression test in patients with mood disorders. J Clin Psychiatry 1996;57:470–84.
91. Berk M, Copolov DL, Dean O, et al. N-acetyl cysteine for depressive symptoms in bipolar disorder–a double-blind randomized placebo-controlled trial. Biol Psychiatry 2008;64:468–75.
92. Berk M, Dean OM, Cotton SM, et al. Maintenance N-acetyl cysteine treatment for bipolar disorder: a double-blind randomized placebo controlled trial. BMC Med 2012;10:91.
93. Nery FG, Monkul ES, Hatch JP, et al. Celecoxib as an adjunct in the treatment of depressive or mixed episodes of bipolar disorder: a double-blind, randomized, placebo-controlled study. Hum Psychopharmacol 2008;23:87–94.
94. Saroukhani S, Emami-Parsa M, Modabbernia A, et al. Aspirin for treatment of lithium-associated sexual dysfunction in men: randomized double-blind placebo-controlled study. Bipolar Disord 2013;15:650–6.
95. Stoll AL, Severus WE, Freeman MP, et al. Omega 3 fatty acids in bipolar disorder: a preliminary double-blind, placebo-controlled trial. Arch Gen Psychiatry 1999;56:407–12.
96. Hirashima F, Parow AM, Stoll AL, et al. Omega-3 fatty acid treatment and T(2) whole brain relaxation times in bipolar disorder. Am J Psychiatry 2004;161:1922–4.
97. Keck PE Jr, Mintz J, McElroy SL, et al. Double-blind, randomized, placebo-controlled trials of ethyl-eicosapentanoate in the treatment of bipolar depression and rapid cycling bipolar disorder. Biol Psychiatry 2006;60:1020–2.
98. Frangou S, Lewis M, McCrone P. Efficacy of ethyl-eicosapentaenoic acid in bipolar depression: randomised double-blind placebo-controlled study. Br J Psychiatry 2006;188:46–50.
99. Frangou S, Lewis M, Wollard J, et al. Preliminary in vivo evidence of increased N-acetyl-aspartate following eicosapentanoic acid treatment in patients with bipolar disorder. J Psychopharmacol (Oxford, England) 2007;21:435–9.
100. Zeinoddini A, Sorayani M, Hassanzadeh E, et al. Pioglitazone adjunctive therapy for depressive episode of bipolar disorder: a randomized, double-blind, placebo-controlled trial. Depress Anxiety 2015;32:167–73.
101. Savitz J, Preskorn S, Teague TK, et al. Minocycline and aspirin in the treatment of bipolar depression: a protocol for a proof-of-concept, randomised, double-blind, placebo-controlled, 2x2 clinical trial. BMJ Open 2012;2:e000643.
102. Magalhaes PV, Dean OM, Bush AI, et al. N-acetylcysteine for major depressive episodes in bipolar disorder. Rev Bras Psiquiatr 2011;33:374–8.
103. Berk M, Dean O, Cotton SM, et al. The efficacy of N-acetylcysteine as an adjunctive treatment in bipolar depression: an open label trial. J Affect Disord 2011; 135:389–94.
104. Bloch MH, Hannestad J. Omega-3 fatty acids for the treatment of depression: systematic review and meta-analysis. Mol Psychiatry 2012;17:1272–82.
105. Kemp DE, Schinagle M, Gao K, et al. PPAR-gamma agonism as a modulator of mood: proof-of-concept for pioglitazone in bipolar depression. CNS Drugs 2014;28:571–81.
106. Soczynska JK, Mansur RB, Brietzke E, et al. Novel therapeutic targets in depression: minocycline as a candidate treatment. Behav Brain Res 2012;235:302–17.
107. Raison CL, Rutherford RE, Woolwine BJ, et al. A randomized controlled trial of the tumor necrosis factor antagonist infliximab for treatment-resistant depression: the role of baseline inflammatory biomarkers. JAMA Psychiatry 2013;70: 31–41.

Genetics of Bipolar Disorder

Recent Update and Future Directions

Fernando S. Goes, MD

KEYWORDS

- Bipolar disorder • Genetics • GWAS • Sequencing • Copy number variation (CNV)
- Family study • Personalized medicine • Pharmacogenetics

KEY POINTS

- Bipolar disorder (BD) is a disabling, often lifelong, disorder that is among the most highly heritable of all common disorders.
- Ongoing genome-wide association studies (GWAS) are yielding more robustly associated markers; next-generation sequencing technologies are poised to identify of rare and potentially more penetrant variants.
- The modest effect sizes seen among GWAS associations are consistent with a polygenic genetic architecture, with risk being distributed across a large number of loci.
- Future progress in common (GWAS) and rare variant studies will provide novel insights into the biology of BD, and help pave the way for personalized medicine and improved, targeted therapies.

INTRODUCTION

Bipolar disorder (BD) is a lifelong disorder marked by periodic disturbances in mood, cognition and behavior. When strictly defined, it is characterized by the presence of manic episodes with marked changes in mood, energy, and cognition that are often associated with psychotic symptoms. The magnitude or severity of manic episodes can be variable, and milder (hypo)manic episodes can be seen in up to 2% to 3% of the general population.[1] Despite the nosologic emphasis on elevated mood episodes, most of the cumulative morbidity arises from depressive episodes, which occur more often and last longer than the briefer periods of mood elevation. Although descriptions of syndromic alteration in mood states have been present since antiquity,

Disclosures: The author has received research support from the NIMH (R00MH86049). The author has no relevant conflict of interests.

Department of Psychiatry and Behavioral Sciences, Johns Hopkins University School of Medicine, Meyer 4-119A, 600 North Wolfe Street, Baltimore, MD 21212, USA

E-mail address: fgoes1@jhmi.edu

it was Emil Kraepelin who provided an initial "synthesis" of a bewildering variety of pathologic mood states into a single nosologic entity that still forms the basic conception of the modern definitions of BD. Kraepelin's notion of "manic–depressive insanity" included a broad variety of mood states, of variable severity that were linked by a remitting "uniform prognosis" and a "hereditary taint."[2] The latter observation spawned more than a century of genetic research into BD, although it has only been in last several years that clearly replicated findings have emerged, in large part owing to the application of reliable, high-throughput technologies to samples of sufficient size made possible by worldwide collaboration. This review highlights recent findings in the field of BD genetics and looks forward to the potential role that future genetic findings will have on clinical care.

FAMILY STUDIES: MEASURING HERITABILITY FROM THE TOP DOWN

A long line of family studies, beginning from the early 20th century work of Kraepelin's student Ernst Rudin, to the more recent studies based on the *Diagnostic and Statistical Manual of Mental Disorders* in the early 21st century, have found consistent evidence for strong familial aggregation of BD type I, ranging from concordance rates of 40% to 70% in monozygotic twins, to approximately 8% to 10% in first-degree relatives.[3] More recent family studies have made use of nationwide registry data in the Scandinavian countries, which provide essentially the only method to ascertain a comprehensive sample despite the disadvantage of only including subjects with the disorder who have sought clinical care and have been accurately diagnosed.[4,5] A recent study of BD using Swedish registry data has been particularly informative for its consideration of the familial aggregation of BD with all the major psychiatric disorders.[5] Consistent with prior interview-based family studies, Song and colleagues[5] found strong evidence for familial aggregation of BD-I with first-degree relative risks (RR) of 5.8 to 7.9. However, the large sample size provided the statistical power to detect coaggregation of BD and schizophrenia (RR, 2.8), major depression (RR, 2.1), anxiety disorders (RR, 1.8), attention deficit hyperactivity disorder (RR, 2.4), personality disorders (RR, 2.2), autism (RR, 2.6), as well as drug abuse disorders (RR, 1.7). These findings are consistent with the familial transmission of a more generalized increased risk for a broad array of psychopathology, which has also gained support from genome-wide association studies (GWAS).

In contrast, 2 recent interview-based family studies of BD that attempted to ascertain the full spectrum of mood disorders have highlighted the relative independence of BD-I and psychotic disorders from the more common unipolar and anxiety diagnoses.[6,7] Although these studies distinguish themselves from prior interview-based studies by their broader ascertainment and their use of nonhierarchical diagnoses, they may have failed to detect a modest coaggregation with psychotic disorders because of their more limited sample size. Indeed, prior family studies of BD often showed a modest increase in rates of schizophrenia, but because of the difficulties in collecting large numbers of families, they lacked the power to detect a statistically significant difference. However, a recent metaanalysis of 38 family showed evidence for a consistent but modest increase in rates of schizophrenia in first degree family members of subjects with BD (odds ratio [OR], 2.10).[8] Nevertheless, these studies raise the important point that ascertainment and diagnostic assessment (including the emphasis placed on diagnostic hierarchy) is an important factor influencing patterns of familial transmission. Despite highlighting differing conclusions, the overall pattern seen within the broader context of published BD literature is generally consistent: BD-I has the highest RRs among first degree family members (RR ~ 8–10), with far lower familial risks for "other" disorders (RR ~ 2) that range from subthreshold mood and anxiety disorders to psychotic disorders.

What is the relevance of such family studies in an era of increasing molecular sophistication? By relying almost entirely on clinical phenotypes, family studies are subject to the usual criticisms of clinically defined studies based on descriptive syndromes: overlapping symptoms, variable reliability, and uncertain mapping onto an underlying biology. However, although clinical phenotypes remain broad proxies for an elusive underlying biology, they reflect the clinical reality that is most pertinent to patients and clinicians and still provide the most discriminative "index" relevant for clinical decision making. Indeed, because family history is a broad proxy encompassing all transmitted genetic variation as well as shared environment, it remains the single strongest measurable risk factor for development of BD.

MOLECULAR STUDIES: MEASURING HERITABILITY FROM THE BOTTOM UP

Heritability is an estimate of what proportion of a disorder can be attributed to genetic variation, but it provides no guidance on whether the underlying genetic causes are few or many, common or rare, or somewhere in between.[9] The relative contribution of common versus rare variants for psychiatric phenotypes has been a subject of much debate. Fortunately, empirical data are beginning to settle this debate.

Initial approaches to mapping genes for BD were limited by sparse, low-resolution linkage technologies, which could point to a broad area of a chromosome if a disorder was strongly linked to 1 or only few specific regions. Although the genome-wide linkage approach worked well with Mendelian diseases, it has been generally unsuccessful for common diseases that likely consist of more diverse and nuanced genetic causes. Numerous genome-wide linkage studies of BD were performed in the last 2 decades, and the failure to identify a consistent linkage signal is an indication that the more moderately penetrant variants seen in certain complex disorders (such as the MHC locus in autoimmune disorders) are unlikely to be found for BD.[10]

ASSOCIATION STUDIES: SUCCESS OF GENOME-WIDE APPROACHES AT SCALE

After the sequencing of the human genome it became apparent that most genetic variation is composed of single nucleotide polymorphisms, which represent single base-pair changes that occur regularly throughout the genome at approximately every 1000 bases for a total of approximately 3.5 million in a genome.[11] Technological advances led to accurate and cost-effective methods to genotype single nucleotide polymorphisms throughout out the genome in a highly automated assay that has become known as a GWAS. Before GWAS, association studies in BD were limited to 1 or a few genes ("candidate gene studies") and suffered from poor reproducibility owing to small sample sizes and the challenges of selecting candidate genes given the limited knowledge of the pathophysiology of BD. Fortunately, the last decade has seen a transition to genome-wide approaches, which provide an agnostic yet comprehensive approach.

GWAS have now been performed successfully on almost all medically relevant phenotypes and, despite a few exceptions,[12] has led to replicable associations that can provide "entry points" into disease related biology. Importantly, GWAS data are easily compared or metaanalyzed across studies through a process known as imputation, in which common variants in correlation with a known genotype can be probabilistically inferred ("imputed") based on known patterns within the human population. A second important consideration has been the establishment of clear guidelines for considering a finding to be genome-wide significant.[13] Simulation and empirical approaches have demonstrated that the genome has approximately 1 million common independent markers, leading to a corrected association P value threshold of 5×10^{-8} (derived by dividing the conventional $P<.05$ value by approximately 1 million tests).[13] Typically findings that cross this threshold in a primary analysis have a high rate of replication and go on to show genome-wide evidence of association in subsequent metaanalyses.

In most disorders, including psychiatric disorders, initial GWAS samples (consisting of a few thousand cases and controls) were underpowered to detect genome-wide significant associations. This has led to the formation of consortia, such as the Psychiatric GWAS Consortium (PGC), in which large-scale metaanalyses have been performed in sample sizes that now include tens of thousands cases and controls. As sample sizes increase and initial GWAS findings begin to emerge, an "inflection point" is reached where further addition of samples leads to a regular, linear increase in genome-wide significant findings. For example, in schizophrenia, the latest published analysis of 36,989 cases and 113,075 controls is now beyond the "inflection point," with a yield of 108 genome-wide significant loci.[14]

Progress in BD will likely follow a similar pattern, although sample sizes are smaller and the "inflection point" has not yet been reached. The first GWAS of BD consisted of 1868 cases and 2938 controls and was conducted by the Wellcome Trust consortium in 2007.[15] This was followed by several similarly sized studies, with no individual study large enough to identify genome-wide significant findings.[16–19] Yet, as samples began to be metaanalyzed a number of replicated findings have emerged. In 2011 the PGC published its first BD metaanalysis consisting of 11,974 cases and 51,792 controls,[20] finding genome-wide significant evidence in 2 loci within the L-type calcium channel subunit gene *CACNA1C* and the cell surface receptor protein *ODZ4*. Several additional metaanalyses have been published subsequently,[21–24] and their genome-wide significant results are summarized in **Table 1**.

The results shown in **Table 1** show typical characteristic of GWAS findings: (1) most highly associated markers are intronic (ie, within or next to genes but outside of the protein coding region), (2) their effect sizes (OR) are small and all are less than 1.2, and (3) associations are independent of each other, with no statistical evidence for gene–gene interactions. Importantly, owing to the close correlation of markers in nearby regions of the chromosomes, GWAS associations highlight broad genomic regions, known as loci, that can span up to several hundred thousand base pairs. The actual marker that led to the association is generally unlikely to be the "causal" marker within a locus and additional investigation is necessary to uncover the actual genetic variants that have a functional effect.

FROM GENOME-WIDE ASSOCIATION STUDIES TO FUNCTION: ELUCIDATING MECHANISM

Once a genome-wide association is confirmed and replicated in a subsequent metaanalysis, the arguably more challenging task of elucidating the molecular mechanisms behind the association lies ahead.[25] As an example of the type of further evaluation required to link a GWAS loci with its interacting gene(s), Roussos and colleagues[26] performed a comprehensive evaluation of findings from a recently published schizophrenia GWAS that included the same *CACNA1C* locus identified in GWAS metaanalyses of BD (see **Table 1**). The authors identified a number of additional markers in

Table 1

Genome-wide significant loci in bipolar disorder

Nearest Gene	Chr	Marker	Risk Allele	P-value	Odds Ratio	Cases (N)	Controls (N)	Study
Loci with initial genome-wide significant evidence ($P < 5 \times 10^{-8}$) and at least one additional replication								
TRANK1	3p22	rs9834970	C	2.4×10^{-11}	1.18	6,658	7,155	Chen et al,[22] 2011
				4.8×10^{-8}	1.12	9,747	14,278	Muhleisen et al,[24] 2014
ANK3	10q21	rs10994415	C	6.9×10^{-11}	1.27	9,747	14,278	Muhleisen et al,[24] 2014
ODZ4	11q14	rs12576775	A	4.4×10^{-8}	0.88	11,974	51,792	PGC-BD et al,[20] 2011
				6.2×10^{-9}	0.88	13,192	54,705	Green et al,[23] 2013
				4.5×10^{-9}	0.85	9,747	14,278	Muhleisen et al,[24] 2014
CACNA1C	12p13	rs4765913	A	1.5×10^{-8}	1.14	11,974	51,792	PGC-BD et al,[20] 2011
				9.8×10^{-10}	1.14	13,192	54,705	Green et al,[23] 2013
NCAN	19p13	rs1064395	A	2.1×10^{-9}	1.17	7,759	34,062	Cichon et al,[21] 2011
Loci with initial genome-wide significant evidence ($P < 5 \times 10^{-8}$)								
RHEBL1/DHH	12q13	rs7296288	A	9.0×10^{-9}	0.90	13,192	54,705	Green et al,[23] 2013
TRPC4AP	20q11	rs3818253	A	3.9×10^{-8}	1.16	8,699	12,163	Green et al,[23] 2013
ADCY2	5p15	rs17826816	G	9.9×10^{-9}	1.14	9,747	14,278	Muhleisen et al,[24] 2014
MIR2113; POU3F2	6q16	rs12202969	A	1.1×10^{-8}	1.12	9,747	14,278	Muhleisen et al,[24] 2014
PTGFR	1p31	rs4650608	T	8.4×10^{-9}	0.88	7,773	9,883	Chen et al,[22] 2011
LMAN2L	2q11	rs2271893	G	5.2×10^{-9}	0.86	7,773	9,883	Chen et al,[22] 2011
Many genes	3p21	rs7618915	G	1.6×10^{-9}	0.87	7,773	9,883	Chen et al,[22] 2011
SYNE1	6q25	rs9371601	T	2.9×10^{-8}	1.10	9,368	10,929	Green et al,[74] 2013

Loci with subsequent evidence for replication in an independent sample are shown in the top part of the table, while loci with initial evidence for genome-wide significance only are shown in the bottom of the table. Although studies are listed independently, there is substantial overlap among the cases and controls between the studies.

Data from Refs.[20–24,74]

strong correlation with the index marker in regions known as enhancers that regulate the transcription of a nearby gene. The marker associated with BD and schizophrenia was shown subsequently to be associated with decreased enhancer binding to the promoter of *CACNA1C* and lower levels of transcription.[26] These experiments involved the use of post mortem brain tissue, neural progenitor cells, and nonneural cell lines, reflecting the need for a comprehensive approach to functional validation of a GWAS loci, particularly for psychiatric disorders where not all tissues or cell lines may be equally relevant.

Historically, the main source of human neural tissue has been post mortem brain samples, which are limited by well known confounds such as differential environmental exposures and post mortem related artifacts. As a result, there has been a widespread embracement of novel cellular reprograming technologies that can transform somatic cells (obtained from skin or blood) into neural progenitor cell lines or lineage specific neural cell lines.[27] Although this remains a nascent field, particularly in its application to complex brain disorders, the use of transformed neural cells is likely to provide a feasible and relevant model system to study important aspects of neural physiology. Only a few initial stem cell studies have been performed with BD,[28–30] with preliminary results of the most comprehensive study indicating that BD may be associated with a hyperexcitable neuronal phenotype that is differentially responsive to lithium in subjects successfully treated with lithium.[30] If confirmed, such cellular phenotypes may show promise as potential biomarkers of clinical response and may provide a means for high-throughput testing of the biological effects of newly discovered genetic variants and novel therapeutic compounds.

Of course, gene expression is only the most initial "downstream" phenotype and establishing a causal chain from genome to the ultimate (clinical) phenotype will require studying the effects of an associated locus on protein, cell, and ultimately physiologic function. Elucidating how a putative disease related biological effect is "transmitted" across such increasingly complex hierarchies of biological processes will be a major focus of research for the conceivable future.[31] Imaging modalities will no doubt play an increasingly important role, although most current studies are hindered by small sample size and limited interstudy comparability.[32] Fortunately, the technological innovations and large-scale consortia that were integral to the success of genetic studies are also now occurring in the field of imaging and imaging genetics.[33,34]

Polygenic Risk Scores

In addition to the few associations that meet the stringent level for genome-wide significance, a GWAS study will have a much greater number of associated markers that do not meet genome-wide significance. Although the confidence that any 1 such marker is associated with the studied phenotype is low, these subthreshold markers can be grouped to create a polygenic "signature" that is highly reproducible across GWAS datasets and can account for a much higher proportion of the phenotypic variation compared with any individual marker.[35] The magnitude of the polygenic association generally depends on the power of the initial "training" dataset from which the subthreshold associations are derived. Because power in a GWAS study correlates strongly with sample size, increasing the sample size of disorder-specific GWAS will lead to predictable improvements in the ability of polygenic scores to discriminate cases from controls. For example, in the schizophrenia PGC2 study, the polygenic score was associated with approximately 10% to 20% of the phenotypic variance in an independent sample.[14] The smaller BD training dataset so far yields a more modest, but still highly significant, association that accounts for approximately 3% of the phenotypic variance.[20]

Another important use of polygenic scores is that they can be used to model the proportion of the overall heritability that can be attributed to common variants. The development of analytical methods that measure the overall proportion of shared common variation throughout the genome in cases versus controls has provided estimates that at least 25% of the overall heritability of BD can be explained by common variants.[36] This estimate provides a strong impetus to increase GWAS sample sizes, because the currently discovered genome-wide significant findings explain no more than a few percent of the overall heritability.

A more elusive goal is the application of polygenic scores for phenotype prediction. Currently available scores, for either schizophrenia or BD, explain far too little of the phenotypic variance to be clinically meaningful by themselves, with prediction area under the curve estimates no greater than approximately 0.6.[37] However, under "optimal" conditions, when polygenic scores can be estimated from extremely large discovery samples (at least an order of magnitude greater than currently available samples), clinical utility may be achievable with potential under the curve values in the 0.8 to 0.9 range.[38] One important caveat is that even the perfect genetic test will be constrained by the overall heritability of BD (≈ 0.7). Hence, the most informative type of test will also likely need to incorporate other markers or "proxies" of pathophysiological or environmental states to provide further predictive capacity.

Although the prospects for clinical prediction lie in the future, polygenic scores are currently of research interest as an index of genetic liability to a specific disorder. In a recent study of schizophrenia, for example, family history was found to interact with polygenic scores to increase the risk of schizophrenia,[39] pointing to the need for further studies to characterize important elements of family history that are both dependent and independent of genetic liability. More broadly, this type of analysis can also be used to better characterize the genetic effects on clinically relevant phenotypes, such as illness course and drug response, which are likely to be better predicted by polygenic rather than single marker models.

Rare Variants: The Next Frontier

Genetic variation can be arbitrarily defined as rare if it is present in less than 1% of a studied sample or population. Rare variation may be particularly relevant for the understanding of disease related biology, because rare variants are evolutionarily more recent and have had less time to be selected against or removed by evolution.[40] Hence, rare variants may be more likely to be pathogenic compared with common variants and could therefore provide a more direct and actionable insight into disease pathophysiology.[41] Highly penetrant rare variants are responsible for most Mendelian disorders and, although such strongly associated variants have not been found for most psychiatric disorders, the identification of variants with penetrance in between those responsible for Mendelian disorders and those found by GWAS is currently a major focus of research.

Copy Number Variants

A recently described type of variation that arises from subtle misalignment errors during DNA repair and replication is known as a copy number variation (CNV) and consists of large deletions or duplications of several thousand to a million base pairs. For much the same reasons described previously, rare CNVs tend to be more pathogenic than common CNVs, especially larger CNVs, which are more likely to disrupt a single gene or a group of genes. Rare CNVs were first found to be overrepresented in cases with early onset neurodevelopmental disorders such as autism and intellectual disability.[42]

Table 2
Copy number variations (CNV) nominal significance (P<.05) for association with BD

CNV Locus	Odds Ratio[a]	P-Value	Frequency Cases	Frequency Controls
1q21.1 duplication	2.6	.02	0.099% (8/8084)	0.037% (24/64,046)
3q29 deletion	17.3	.03	0.025% (2/8084)	0.0014% (1/69,965)
16p11.2 duplication	4.4	2.3×10^{-4}	0.13% (12/9129)	0.03% (19/63,068)

Abbreviation: CNV, copy number variation.
[a] Effect estimates and raw numbers obtained from the meta-analysis performed by Green and colleagues.
Data from Green EK, Rees E, Walters JT et al. Copy number variation in bipolar disorder. Mol Psychiatry 2015;[Epub ahead of print].

Subsequent studies have expanded the range of disorders affected by CNVs to include adult onset disorders such as schizophrenia[43] and, to a lesser extent, BD.[44,45]

In a recent study of BD that also collated findings from the literature, Georgieva and colleagues[44] reported significantly increased risk of de novo CNVs in BD, when defining a CNV as any deletion or duplication greater than 10 kilobases (crude OR, 2.2; P = .0003). Although they also found a trend toward increased risk for larger (greater than 100 kilobases) de novo CNVs, this difference was not statistically significant (crude OR, 1.46; P = .18). Compared with schizophrenia, the association of de novo CNV variants with BD seems to be more modest in both the magnitude of the association and the actual size of the CNV. A similar pattern is seen in case-control studies of CNVs where most of the discovered CNVs consist of inherited, rather than de novo CNVs.[45] **Table 2** highlights the findings of a recent large scale study and meta-analysis of CNVs in BD, which found the most consistent evidence for the association of 3 recurrent CNVs with BD, with the strongest findings seen with the 16p11.2 duplication. The CNV associations shown in **Table 2** share a number of important characteristics: (1) The effect size of the associations are much higher compared with common variants; (2) All CNVs have also been found in controls, albeit at a much lower frequency; (3) Each CNV is associated with multiple genes; (4) Each CNV is individually rare and collectively affect only approximately 0.3% of all cases; and (5) All highlighted CNVs have also been associated more strongly with schizophrenia.

Next-Generation Sequencing

Most rare variation, like most common variation, is composed of single nucleotide changes or deletions. Yet, because rare variation is poorly represented in GWAS arrays, the only comprehensive means of assessing its role in disease susceptibility is by DNA sequencing. Fortunately, recent technological advances have changed the feasibility of large scale DNA sequencing, with whole genomes now routinely sequenced in several days for approximately $1000. Two major assays are used to measure rare variants in clinical and research settings: whole genome sequencing and a more targeted form of sequencing known as whole exome sequencing, which is limited to the approximately 1.5% of the genome that is transcribed into messenger RNA and translated into protein. Whole exome sequencing has the advantage of lower cost, a lower bioinformatic "footprint," and a focus on the more easily interpretable part of the genome where most variants responsible for Mendelian disorders have been identified to date.[46] However, whole exome sequencing misses variation in the noncoding (including regulatory) regions and is less accurate in detecting important types of variations such as insertions, deletions, or CNVs. Although whole exome sequencing is currently the most widely used genetic assay of rare variants, it will ultimately be supplanted by whole genome sequencing as sequencing costs decrease.

The role of rare sequence variation in psychiatric disorders is an active area of research, with particular emphasis on the study of more heritable syndromes such as intellectual disability, autism, schizophrenia, and BD. In a pattern similar to that seen in the CNV studies, the effect of rare variants—particularly de novo rare variants—seem to be more prominent in neurodevelopmental disorders, such as intellectual disability or certain forms of autism, where gene-disrupting mutations have been found to cluster in pathways involved in transcriptional regulation and synaptic function.[47,48] In schizophrenia, a recent exome sequencing study of 623 trios did not implicate a specific gene, but found enrichment of rare de novo variants in pathways associated with the postsynaptic density.[49] A complementary exome case-control study of schizophrenia[49] showed similar enrichment for very rare mutations in postsynaptic gene sets (in particular, the activity-regulated cytoskeleton-associated protein and N-methyl-D-aspartate receptor gene sets), as well as in calcium channel subunits, which had been previously implicated in the PGC2 GWAS study.

A number of BD sequencing studies are ongoing, but only a few family-based sequencing studies have been published so far.[50–54] Two of these studies have included Amish samples, including the exceptionally large pedigree first described by Egeland and colleagues[55] in 1987. However, the investigators were unable to find rare pathogenic variants that segregated in most affected family members, leading them to conclude that genetic heterogeneity may be present even within a family.[51] The results of these initial studies have so far not shown clear convergence on a specific gene, although larger and more comprehensive analyses are currently under way within the Bipolar Sequencing Consortium. At the same time, a number of research groups are also performing exome or whole genome sequencing of large case-control samples, with results expected in early 2016. Together, these case-control studies should have sufficient sample size (several thousand cases and controls) to identify what may be considered "low-hanging fruit." Ongoing studies of other complex disorders with similar samples sizes have identified significant enrichment of rare-variants within genes in certain disorders like amyotrophic lateral sclerosis[56]; however, the study of most other complex disorders has not yet led to significant findings, indicating the need for larger samples sizes likely in the range of 10 to 20,000 cases.[57]

Genetic Architecture of Bipolar Disease

The overall number of risk alleles, their individual frequency, and their effect sizes is collectively referred to as the genetic architecture of a particular phenotype or trait. Although significant heritability implies that genetics plays a causal role in disease, the actual genetic architecture underlying the heritability cannot be predicted and needs to be determined empirically. At 1 extreme are many of the classically Mendelian disorders, where only 1 very rare and penetrant type of mutation can account for the entire disease phenotype. At the other extreme are disorders with prominent polygenicity, marked by a very large number (several hundreds or thousands) of risk alleles that individually increases risk modestly but collectively account for most of the heritability. The gap between the heritability predicted from twin and family studies and the heritability explained by identified variants has been termed the "missing heritability." Yet, as Witte and colleagues[37] have commented, much of it should be considered "hidden" rather than "missing" because increasing samples for both GWAS and rare variants studies should in the near future explain a significant amount of this hidden heritability, as is occurring in other complex phenotypes such as height, Crohn's disease, and body mass index.

Fig. 1 shows where the current findings described in this article fall on the genomic architecture space, with relatively high effect sizes seen for the rare CNV mutations, compared with the much lower effects sizes seen for the more common GWAS associations. Although the number of robustly confirmed loci remains relatively small, sample sizes in BD have only just reached the numbers where most complex disorders begin to yield findings in a predictable incremental manner. By early 2016, the PGC metaanalysis is expected to include more than 35,000 BD cases, which is equivalent to the sample size that yielded more than 100 genome-wide significant findings for schizophrenia. Consequently, it is reasonable to assume that the number of common variants associated with BD will increase rapidly over the next year.

The near term results for rare variants is perhaps more uncertain, because the methodology is newer and the number of samples with whole exome or genome sequencing is still much less than that available for GWAS. Available data from other complex disorders along with theoretically based simulations suggest that, like GWAS, sample sizes will likely need to be in the tens of thousands to begin yielding significant findings at realistic effect sizes.[58] The next several years should reveal whether more penetrant mutations exist in BD, as has been found in autism and intellectual disability. Although there are evolutionary reasons to believe that rare variants of large effect are more likely to be found in early onset disorders with low fecundity,[59] this does not diminish the potential importance of identifying even a

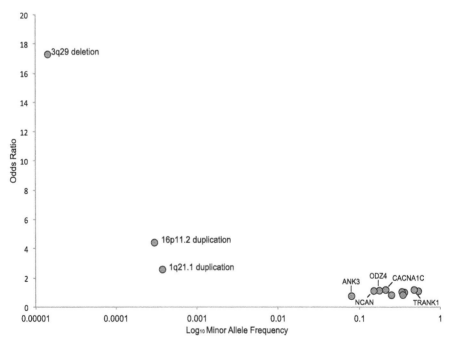

Fig. 1. Emerging genetic architecture of bipolar disorder. Risk loci are show in relationship to their effect size (y axis) and their frequency in control populations (x axis). Loci represent those shown in Tables 1 and 2. For the common variants, only those with genome-wide significant evidence for replication and additional replication are labeled with text. (Data from Refs.[20–24,45,74])

relatively small number of rare but highly penetrant variants, because such variants can yield almost immediate insights into disease biology and identify novel therapeutic targets. There are now several successful examples of very rare variants of high effect that have identified therapeutic targets, including the recently approved PCSK-9 inhibitors for hyperlipidemia.[60]

Blurring of Diagnostic Boundaries: Cross-Disorder Associations

A major feature of many of the discovered genetic associations with BD has been their concurrent associations with other phenotypes, particularly schizophrenia. For example, 4 of the genome-wide significant variants shown in **Table 1** (within or near the genes *TRANK1*, *CACNA1C*, *NCAN*, and the multigenic 3p21 locus) were also found to be genome-wide significant in the PCG2 GWAS of schizophrenia.[14] In addition, all the rare CNVs shown in **Table 2** have also been found in CNV studies of schizophrenia.[42] Interestingly, the rare CNV variants also show overlap with studies of autism, a phenotype for which the rare variants have thus far been studied more intensively than common variants. Prominent overlap is also present among the many subthreshold common associations that drive cross-disorder polygenic risk associations across most major psychiatric disorders, with a particularly strong genetic correlation (GWAS based correlation of 0.68) between BD and schizophrenia.[36]

At a genome-wide level, these correlations reflect a widely seen property of individual or aggregated variants, both common and rare, known as pleiotropy, which in its simplest definition is the association of a genetic risk factor with more than 1 trait.[61] Pleiotropy is a phenomenon widely seen across species, reflecting the many potential ways to affect a phenotype in the long complex causal chain between a gene and the observable trait of interest. At a broad level, potential factors involved in pleiotropy may include differing gene–gene interactions (including the effect of the overall genomic background), developmental effects, and differential environmental effects, which are all areas of active scientific investigation.

These correlations complement the results seen from the more recent population-based studies,[4,5] and have important implications for psychiatry nosology, largely confirming long-held suspicions that the diagnostic borders across phenotypes may not reflect biological boundaries.[62] However, it must also be emphasized that their specific relevance for clinical care is still uncertain, because the relationship of polygenic risk scores to clinically relevant phenotypes such as prognosis and treatment response remains an area of active investigation.

Pharmacogenetics

Potentially the most clinically relevant application of genetics to patients with BD may arise from the field of pharmacogenetics, which investigates how genetic variation affects both the efficacy and metabolism of therapeutic drugs. Because it is less likely that variants associated with drug response or drug tolerability have been under negative evolutionary pressure, there are theoretical reasons to expect that pharmacogenetics variants may have larger effect sizes and be more clinically actionable. Indeed, in other fields of medicine, a number of high-effect variants have been identified in a wide variety of drug response studies that range from efficacy of interferon treatment in hepatitis C to the dosing of anticoagulants.[63] Most identified variants have been related to drug metabolism and adverse side effects rather than therapeutic effect, presumably reflecting the more complex nature of the latter.

In BD, initial investigations have focused on the response to mood stabilizers, particularly lithium.[64] One difficulty of such studies is the appropriate measure of the drug response phenotype, which usually requires a substantial longitudinal component and careful attention to common confounders like the use of additional medications, illicit drug use, and variable medication adherence. Not surprisingly, most published studies have been limited by small sample sizes and prominent inter-study heterogeneity. A number of candidate gene studies have been published and, although some have shown evidence for replication, the overall level of evidence remains modest and below that of the previously described disease-specific GWAS findings.[65]

To date, there have been 3 GWAS of lithium response and no such studies of response to other BD medications. The first lithium response GWAS was a secondary analysis using longitudinal data from the STEP-BD trial (up to 2 years of follow-up) to characterize the association between common variants and relapse in 458 subjects on lithium treatment.[66] The authors did not find any genome-wide significant findings, but attempted to replicate their top results in an independent case-control sample using a retrospective measure of lithium response. Five markers showed modest evidence for replication, which included the GluR2 glutamate receptor and *ODZ4*, a gene previously found to be a BD risk gene (see **Table 1**). A more recent study from Taiwan, however, reported an unusually strong association with a marker in glutamate decarboxylase-like protein 1 (*GADL1*), with an effect size (OR, 73.9) that is almost 2 orders of magnitude greater than those seen in any BD case-control GWAS.[67] Although the original study authors also presented consistent replication in an additional sample, a number of failed replications have also been published.[68,69] Hence, the relevance of this finding remains uncertain and in need for further confirmation. The largest and most recent study of lithium response included 2,563 patients collected by the Consortium for Lithium Genetics and phenotyped using a uniform retrospective lithium rating scale.[70] This study found a genome-wide significant association on a locus on chromosome 21 that encompasses two long non-coding RNAs (lncRNAs), which are sequences of DNA that are actively transcribed and may have important roles in the regulation of gene-expression. However, further replication is needed and additional work is required to determine whether any potential causal relationship between the associated markers and the expression of lncRNAs.[70] With the exception of the unusually large effect finding from the Taiwanese study, these initial GWAS show the more typical modest effect sizes that require large samples sizes and also point to the likelihood that lithium response may also be a complex, polygenic phenotype.

Toward Personalized Medicine

As a disorder defined at the level of syndrome, with prominent heterogeneity at the level of clinical symptoms, long-term outcome, and response to treatment, BD is long due some element of personalization. The goals of personalized medicine are not new, but the recent widespread availability of genomic and other "-omic" based technologies, along with availability of large-scale cohorts, has renewed focus on identifying novel ways to classify patients and help identify treatments targeted to a specific disease related pathophysiology.

For clinicians treating patients with BD, there are a number of well-known clinical dilemmas to be (re)addressed in this new era of personalized or precision medicine. First, there is a need for improved prediction of BD in the prodromal years when children and adolescents suffer primarily from a broad range of subthreshold mood, anxiety, and behavioral disorders before the emergence of (hypo)mania.[71] Second, the course of BD can differ widely between patients, with marked heterogeneity in terms of initial episode polarity, recurrence, association with comorbid syndromes, and cognitive impairment.[72] Finally, the most desired outcome of the precision medicine initiative will be to help tailor treatment to patients based on their individual risk factors.

What role will genetics play in these precision medicine goals? To quote a prominent geneticist, "Genetics alone cannot tell us why we are the way we are, but it has a seat at the table."[73] How direct the influence of genetic risk factors will be on clinically relevant phenotypes will be determined by the underlying genetic architecture. If psychiatric disorders are primarily polygenic, then genetics will play a more probabilistic rather than deterministic role in prediction of clinical outcomes, much in the way that certain laboratory tests aid physicians in "risk stratification." For the small minority of patients or families for whom a "simpler" genetic architecture is responsible for their disorder (eg, a rare patient who carries a penetrant CNV mutation), genetics is likely to play a more strongly informative role, but it is currently unclear for what proportion of patients with BD this will be applicable. However, even in such scenarios, because the heritability of BD is less than 100%, nongenetic factors will also play an important role in the manifestation of clinically relevant phenotypes. Elucidation of such factors, which fall under the overly vague label of "environmental" causes, is perhaps a greater challenge than genomics, but it is one that must be addressed to fulfill the promises of personalized medicine.

SUMMARY

The study of genetic factors associated with BD can be safely said to have entered a mature phase, with the appropriate capacity to begin to provide the long awaited insights into the pathophysiology of BD. These advances have been made possible by technological innovations such as large-scale microarray genotyping and next generation sequencing, which have been applied in a comprehensive genome-wide manner to large samples. Several genes have now been robustly associated with BD and in 2016 analyses by the PGC are expected to yield many more similar findings. The initial fruits of such efforts will be to identify molecular targets and pathways that provide insights into the underlying biology of BD and thereby facilitate novel drug development. Eventually, as the field progresses and a greater proportion of heritability is accounted for, more immediate clinical applications such as risk stratification and biologically informed drug selection may also become feasible. However, to keep pace with the technological advances, there is a pressing need now for clinical care to "partner" with research and provide both the samples sizes and the relevant phenotypes necessary to fulfill the promise of precision medicine.

ACKNOWLEDGMENTS

The author thanks the valuable assistance of David Liebers, MPhil, in performing the literature review.

REFERENCES

1. Merikangas KR, Jin R, He JP, et al. Prevalence and correlates of bipolar spectrum disorder in the world mental health survey initiative. Arch Gen Psychiatry 2011; 68(3):241–51.
2. Kraepelin E. Manic-depressive insanity and paranoia. Translated by R. Mary Barclay from the eighth German edition of the 'Textbook of Psychiatry'. Edinburgh: E. & S. Livingstone; 1921.

3. Smoller JW, Finn CT. Family, twin, and adoption studies of bipolar disorder. Am J Med Genet C Semin Med Genet 2003;123C(1):48–58.
4. Mortensen PB, Pedersen CB, Melbye M, et al. Individual and familial risk factors for bipolar affective disorders in Denmark. Arch Gen Psychiatry 2003;60(12): 1209–15.
5. Song J, Bergen SE, Kuja-Halkola R, et al. Bipolar disorder and its relation to major psychiatric disorders: a family-based study in the Swedish population. Bipolar Disord 2014;17(2):184–93.
6. Merikangas KR, Cui L, Heaton L, et al. Independence of familial transmission of mania and depression: results of the NIMH family study of affective spectrum disorders. Mol Psychiatry 2014;19(2):214–9.
7. Vandeleur CL, Merikangas KR, Strippoli MP, et al. Specificity of psychosis, mania and major depression in a contemporary family study. Mol Psychiatry 2014;19(2): 209–13.
8. Van Snellenberg JX, de Candia T. Meta-analytic evidence for familial coaggregation of schizophrenia and bipolar disorder. Arch Gen Psychiatry 2009;66(7):748–55.
9. Visscher PM, Hill WG, Wray NR. Heritability in the genomics era–concepts and misconceptions. Nat Rev Genet 2008;9(4):255–66.
10. Badner JA, Koller D, Foroud T, et al. Genome-wide linkage analysis of 972 bipolar pedigrees using single-nucleotide polymorphisms. Mol Psychiatry 2012;17(8): 818–26.
11. 1000 Genomes Project Consortium, Abecasis GR, Auton A, Brooks LD, et al. An integrated map of genetic variation from 1,092 human genomes. Nature 2012; 491(7422):56–65.
12. Levinson DF, Mostafavi S, Milaneschi Y, et al. Genetic studies of major depressive disorder: why are there no genome-wide association study findings and what can we do about it? Biol Psychiatry 2014;76(7):510–2.
13. McCarthy MI, Abecasis GR, Cardon LR, et al. Genome-wide association studies for complex traits: consensus, uncertainty and challenges. Nat Rev Genet 2008; 9(5):356–69.
14. Schizophrenia Working Group of the Psychiatric Genomics Consortium, Ripke S, Neale BM, Corvin A, et al. Biological insights from 108 schizophrenia-associated genetic loci. Nature 2014;511(7510):421–7.
15. Wellcome Trust Case Control Consortium, Burton PR, Clayton DG, Cardon LR, et al. Genome-wide association study of 14,000 cases of seven common diseases and 3,000 shared controls. Nature 2007;447(7145):661–78.
16. Baum AE, Akula N, Cabanero M, et al. A genome-wide association study implicates diacylglycerol kinase eta (DGKH) and several other genes in the etiology of bipolar disorder. Mol Psychiatry 2008;13(2):197–207.
17. Sklar P, Smoller JW, Fan J, et al. Whole-genome association study of bipolar disorder. Mol Psychiatry 2008;13(6):558–69.
18. Smith EN, Bloss CS, Badner JA, et al. Genome-wide association study of bipolar disorder in European American and African American individuals. Mol Psychiatry 2009;14(8):755–63.
19. Scott LJ, Muglia P, Kong XQ, et al. Genome-wide association and meta-analysis of bipolar disorder in individuals of European ancestry. Proc Natl Acad Sci U S A 2009;106(18):7501–6.
20. Psychiatric GWAS Consortium Bipolar Disorder Working Group, Sklar P, Ripke S, Scott LJ, et al. Large-scale genome-wide association analysis of bipolar disorder identifies a new susceptibility locus near ODZ4. Nat Genet 2011; 43(10):977–83.

21. Cichon S, Muhleisen TW, Degenhardt FA, et al. Genome-wide association study identifies genetic variation in neurocan as a susceptibility factor for bipolar disorder. Am J Hum Genet 2011;88(3):372–81.

22. Chen DT, Jiang X, Akula N, et al. Genome-wide association study meta-analysis of European and Asian-ancestry samples identifies three novel loci associated with bipolar disorder. Mol Psychiatry 2011;18(2):195–205.

23. Green EK, Hamshere M, Forty L, et al. Replication of bipolar disorder susceptibility alleles and identification of two novel genome-wide significant associations in a new bipolar disorder case-control sample. Mol Psychiatry 2013;18(12):1302–7.

24. Muhleisen TW, Leber M, Schulze TG, et al. Genome-wide association study reveals two new risk loci for bipolar disorder. Nat Commun 2014;5:3339.

25. Chakravarti A, Clark AG, Mootha VK. Distilling pathophysiology from complex disease genetics. Cell 2013;155(1):21–6.

26. Roussos P, Mitchell AC, Voloudakis G, et al. A role for noncoding variation in schizophrenia. Cell Rep 2014;9(4):1417–29.

27. Brennand KJ, Simone A, Tran N, et al. Modeling psychiatric disorders at the cellular and network levels. Mol Psychiatry 2012;17(12):1239–53.

28. Chen HM, DeLong CJ, Bame M, et al. Transcripts involved in calcium signaling and telencephalic neuronal fate are altered in induced pluripotent stem cells from bipolar disorder patients. Transl Psychiatry 2014;4:e375.

29. Madison JM, Zhou F, Nigam A, et al. Characterization of bipolar disorder patient-specific induced pluripotent stem cells from a family reveals neurodevelopmental and mRNA expression abnormalities. Mol Psychiatry 2015;20(6):703–17.

30. Mertens J, Wang QW, Kim Y, et al. Differential responses to lithium in hyperexcitable neurons from patients with bipolar disorder. Nature 2015;527(7576):95–9.

31. Insel TR, Cuthbert BN. Medicine. Brain disorders? Precisely. Science 2015; 348(6234):499–500.

32. Savitz JB, Rauch SL, Drevets WC. Clinical application of brain imaging for the diagnosis of mood disorders: the current state of play. Mol Psychiatry 2013; 18(5):528–39.

33. Jorgenson LA, Newsome WT, Anderson DJ, et al. The BRAIN Initiative: developing technology to catalyse neuroscience discovery. Philos Trans R Soc Lond B Biol Sci 2015;370(1668). http://dx.doi.org/10.1098/rstb.2014.0164.

34. Hibar DP, Stein JL, Renteria ME, et al. Common genetic variants influence human subcortical brain structures. Nature 2015;520(7546):224–9.

35. Wray NR, Lee SH, Mehta D, et al. Research review: polygenic methods and their application to psychiatric traits. J Child Psychol Psychiatry 2014;55(10):1068–87.

36. Cross-Disorder Group of the Psychiatric Genomics Consortium, Lee SH, Ripke S, Neale BM, et al. Genetic relationship between five psychiatric disorders estimated from genome-wide SNPs. Nat Genet 2013;45(9):984–94.

37. Witte JS, Visscher PM, Wray NR. The contribution of genetic variants to disease depends on the ruler. Nat Rev Genet 2014;15(11):765–76.

38. Dudbridge F. Power and predictive accuracy of polygenic risk scores. PLoS Genet 2013;9(3):e1003348.

39. Agerbo E, Sullivan PF, Vilhjalmsson BJ, et al. Polygenic risk score, parental socioeconomic status, family history of psychiatric disorders, and the risk for schizophrenia: a Danish population-based study and meta-analysis. JAMA Psychiatry 2015;72(7):635–41.

40. Tennessen JA, Bigham AW, O'Connor TD, et al. Evolution and functional impact of rare coding variation from deep sequencing of human exomes. Science 2012; 337(6090):64–9.

41. Lupski JR, Belmont JW, Boerwinkle E, et al. Clan genomics and the complex architecture of human disease. Cell 2011;147(1):32–43.
42. Malhotra D, Sebat J. CNVs: harbingers of a rare variant revolution in psychiatric genetics. Cell 2012;148(6):1223–41.
43. Kirov G, Pocklington AJ, Holmans P, et al. De novo CNV analysis implicates specific abnormalities of postsynaptic signalling complexes in the pathogenesis of schizophrenia. Mol Psychiatry 2012;17(2):142–53.
44. Georgieva L, Rees E, Moran JL, et al. De novo CNVs in bipolar affective disorder and schizophrenia. Hum Mol Genet 2014;23(24):6677–83.
45. Green EK, Rees E, Walters JT, et al. Copy number variation in bipolar disorder. Mol Psychiatry 2015. [Epub ahead of print].
46. Cirulli ET, Goldstein DB. Uncovering the roles of rare variants in common disease through whole-genome sequencing. Nat Rev Genet 2010;11(6):415–25.
47. Iossifov I, O'Roak BJ, Sanders SJ, et al. The contribution of de novo coding mutations to autism spectrum disorder. Nature 2014;515(7526):216–21.
48. De Rubeis S, He X, Goldberg AP, et al. Synaptic, transcriptional and chromatin genes disrupted in autism. Nature 2014;515(7526):209–15.
49. Fromer M, Pocklington AJ, Kavanagh DH, et al. De novo mutations in schizophrenia implicate synaptic networks. Nature 2014;506(7487):179–84.
50. Collins AL, Kim Y, Szatkiewicz JP, et al. Identifying bipolar disorder susceptibility loci in a densely affected pedigree. Mol Psychiatry 2012;18(12):1245–6.
51. Georgi B, Craig D, Kember RL, et al. Genomic view of bipolar disorder revealed by whole genome sequencing in a genetic isolate. PLoS Genet 2014;10(3): e1004229.
52. Strauss KA, Markx S, Georgi B, et al. A population-based study of KCNH7 p.Arg394His and bipolar spectrum disorder. Hum Mol Genet 2014;23(23): 6395–406.
53. Cruceanu C, Ambalavanan A, Spiegelman D, et al. Family-based exome-sequencing approach identifies rare susceptibility variants for lithium-responsive bipolar disorder. Genome 2013;56(10):634–40.
54. Ament SA, Szelinger S, Glusman G, et al. Rare variants in neuronal excitability genes influence risk for bipolar disorder. Proc Natl Acad Sci U S A 2015; 112(11):3576–81.
55. Egeland JA, Gerhard DS, Pauls DL, et al. Bipolar affective disorders linked to DNA markers on chromosome 11. Nature 1987;325(6107):783–7.
56. Cirulli ET, Lasseigne BN, Petrovski S, et al. Exome sequencing in amyotrophic lateral sclerosis identifies risk genes and pathways. Science 2015;347(6229): 1436–41.
57. Zuk O, Schaffner SF, Samocha K, et al. Searching for missing heritability: designing rare variant association studies. Proc Natl Acad Sci U S A 2014; 111(4):E455–64.
58. Kiezun A, Garimella K, Do R, et al. Exome sequencing and the genetic basis of complex traits. Nat Genet 2012;44(6):623–30.
59. Agarwala V, Flannick J, Sunyaev S, et al. Evaluating empirical bounds on complex disease genetic architecture. Nat Genet 2013;45(12):1418–27.
60. Plenge RM, Scolnick EM, Altshuler D. Validating therapeutic targets through human genetics. Nat Rev Drug Discov 2013;12(8):581–94.
61. Solovieff N, Cotsapas C, Lee PH, et al. Pleiotropy in complex traits: challenges and strategies. Nat Rev Genet 2013;14(7):483–95.
62. Kendell RE. Diagnosis and classification of functional psychoses. Br Med Bull 1987;43(3):499–513.

63. Sala R, Strober MA, Axelson DA, et al. Effects of comorbid anxiety disorders on the longitudinal course of pediatric bipolar disorders. J Am Acad Child Adolesc Psychiatry 2014;53(1):72–81.
64. Alda M. Lithium in the treatment of bipolar disorder: pharmacology and pharmacogenetics. Mol Psychiatry 2015;20(6):661–70.
65. Salloum NC, McCarthy MJ, Leckband SG, et al. Towards the clinical implementation of pharmacogenetics in bipolar disorder. BMC Med 2014;12:90.
66. Perlis RH, Smoller JW, Ferreira MA, et al. A genomewide association study of response to lithium for prevention of recurrence in bipolar disorder. Am J Psychiatry 2009;166(6):718–25.
67. Chen CH, Lee CS, Lee MT, et al. Variant GADL1 and response to lithium therapy in bipolar I disorder. N Engl J Med 2014;370(2):119–28.
68. Consortium on Lithium Genetics, Hou L, Heilbronner U, Rietschel M, et al. Variant GADL1 and response to lithium in bipolar I disorder. N Engl J Med 2014;370(19):1857–9.
69. Ikeda M, Kondo K, Iwata N. Variant GADL1 and response to lithium in bipolar I disorder. N Engl J Med 2014;370(19):1856–7.
70. Hou L, Heilbronner U, Degenhardt F, et al. Genetic variants associated with response to lithium treatment in bipolar disorder: a genome-wide association study. The Lancet, in press.
71. Axelson D, Goldstein B, Goldstein T, et al. Diagnostic precursors to bipolar disorder in offspring of parents with bipolar disorder: a longitudinal study. Am J Psychiatry 2015;172(7):638–46.
72. Frank E, Nimgaonkar VL, Phillips ML, et al. All the world's a (clinical) stage: rethinking bipolar disorder from a longitudinal perspective. Mol Psychiatry 2015. http://dx.doi.org/10.1176/appi.ajp.2014.14010035.
73. Olson MV. Human genetic individuality. Annu Rev Genomics Hum Genet 2012;13:1–27.
74. Green EK, Grozeva D, Forty L, et al. Association at SYNE1 in both bipolar disorder and recurrent major depression. Mol Psychiatry 2013;18(5):614–7.

Index

Note: Page numbers of article titles are in **boldface** type.

Psychiatr Clin N Am 39 (2016) 157–163
http://dx.doi.org/10.1016/S0193-953X(15)00132-X
0193-953X/16/$ – see front matter © 2016 Elsevier Inc. All rights reserved.

psych.theclinics.com

Printed and bound by CPI Group (UK) Ltd, Croydon, CR0 4YY

03/10/2024

01040492-0014